Andreas Jopp

VITAMINS
Life's hidden miracle

Disclaimer

Taking supplements or micronutrients should not be an excuse for a poor nutrition. Vitamins, minerals and trace elements can potentially be overdosed. Those taking higher doses or combine several supplements should consult a certified nutritionist or a doctor. Medical advice can only be given by a licensed healthcare professional who has a chance to personally observe and understand your health condition or objective. Supplements are not meant for self-prescription to cure diseases. The information given in this book is solely intended for information and educational purposes and should not be taken for medical advice. Neither the author not the publisher accept any liability for the reader who chose to self-prescribe. While the information has been researched with best knowledge, science and nutritional studies do uncover new insights and thereby the information of this book may become obsolete. Neither the author nor the publisher assume any legal liability or responsibility for the completeness, the usefulness or the future accuracy of the information. By virtue of this Disclaimer and Warning you may not hold us responsible for any adverse effect you suffer and you may not look to us to indemnify you from your own decision to use supplements.

Warnings

Nutritional supplements can produce adverse reactions in some people. They can interact adversely with other supplements and with prescription drugs or can make prescription drugs ineffective or may boost their potency. Women who are pregnant or nursing should discontinue all supplements except as directed by their healthcare providers. If you observe adverse effects stop taking the supplement immediately and contact your healthcare provider. All supplements should be kept out of the reach of infants and children.

Impressum

Publishing House:
Consult Media Verlag
Vorgebirgstr. 27, 50677 Cologne, Germany.

Rights: All rights reserved to Andreas Jopp.

Picture rights

Cover: istock AniDimi; pg 13 Fotalia JBryson; pg 17 Andreas Jopp;

pg 22 Andreas Jopp; pg Andreas Jopp with friendly permission of Heyne Verlag;

pg 27 Fotalia WaveBreakMediaMicro; pg 59 with friendly permission Thieme Verlag;

pg 61 FotaliaRobert Kneschke; pg 79 Fotalia ArtFamily; pg 90 Antje Plewinsky Fotografie

with friendly permissionHeyne Verlag; pg 107 shutterstock ESB Professional;

pg 131 Istock ariwasabi

Translator: Colin McCullough, Thessaloniki, Greece.

Editor: Andreanna Staubly, Cologne, Germany.

Layout and Graphs: Emergency Design . Nina Fricke, Munich, Germany.

Printed by Create Space

First Edition 2012
Second Edition 2018
ISBN 978-1475040876

Andreas Jopp
is a medical journalist, health coach and bestselling author.

- He has published seven books on the topics of protein, vitamins and minerals, omega-3 fats and health, as well as a multimedia programme to quit smoking.
- The books were listed on the non-fction hit lists of German-based magazines Stern and Focus and have been translated into a total of 16 languages.
- He inspires thousands of attendees at his seminars to make the change to a slimmer, happier and fitter lifestyle.
- He is one of the most prominent nutrition and anti-aging-specialists in Germany.

www.jopp-online.com/en
facebook.com/andreasjopp

Contents

Chapter 5: Who Needs Micronutrients?

Chapter 6: Your personal micronutrient program

Appendix

Introduction

Vitamin and mineral deficiency? Does this still exist today? A deficiency in the midst of incredible abundance? Food of all kinds, including fruits and vegetables are offered in abundance in supermarkets in the developed world. Yet are we in affluent societies deficient in vitamins and minerals despite full plates, due to our bad eating habits? In fact, between 40 and 80% of the population are not even getting the absolute minimum of vitamins and minerals that is necessary for good health. This is the sad result of significant surveys which have been conducted with more than 80,000 people in Germany, France and the United States. 90% of the population is deficient in some of these so-called micro-nutrients. Among these micro-nutrients are vitamin D, folate, iodine and selenium in particular.

Nevertheless, the vast majority of the population is convinced that they cover at least their minimum requirement of micronutrients with their normal diet. This misconception leads to serious health consequences: 70% of today's illnesses are classified as "dietary related". This could be avoided. It is in your hands to supply your body with micronutrients, so that your metabolism and immune system can work optimally.

But watch out: an intake at the low minimum requirement end of the spectrum is not synonymous with an optimal intake that would be necessary for cell protection and for a well-functioning immune system. An analysis of today's foods shows how big the loss of micro-nutrients is and how this loss is caused by storage and processing. An optimal intake can barely be achieved with these foods. The micro-nutrient intake that existed during evolution was much higher.

Long-term observations show that the risk for cardiovascular disease and common cancers can be reduced by half if additional antioxidants (vitamin C, vitamin E and selenium) and B-vitamins - especially folate - are supplied. Solving the vitamin D deficiency also reduces the risk of certain cancers and osteoporosis. Extra folate and vitamin B_{12} reduce the risk of developing dementia. So everyone can use antioxidants and vitamins as a long-term insurance policy for their own health!

But even in the short term an optimal supply of micronutrients influences the metabolism and the immune system. How you feel (nerve metabolism), how energetic you are (energy metabolism) and how well your defence system works against infections (immune function) - all depend on the optimal supply of micronutrients that is involved in every metabolic and every immune function. With a deficiency these systems simply work less effectively. Except for high performance athletes and some top executives, only a few experts use the enormous potential of these biocatalysts. Even though your performance and health is your personal capital and competitive advantage in daily life. Health, fitness and performance are directly dependent on an effectively functioning metabolism.

So, it is in your hands if you want to optimize your metabolism and your immune system with micro-nutrients. To do so, however, requires knowledge and facts. In recent years, this knowledge has exploded in the fields of immune-, genetic- and metabolic-research and the developement of sophisticated analytical methods that can penetrate into the remotest areas of the metabolism. Within a few years we have been catapulted out of the Stone Age, into a new era of research on metabolism and immune function.

Your doctor's advice can be misleading. The reason is that diet and vitamins are not studied in depth when you study to become a doctor. Often doctors' knowledge is minimal and completely outdated in this field. However, they are continuously asked for advice in a field that they know next to nothing about. In addition, this kind of nutritional advice is generally not covered by health insurance. Thus advising patients in this topic steals valuable time while a doctor could be making money. Often the given opinion about vitamins is a quick answer like: "it can't hurt to take them" or "Just eat well. That's enough". Usually to cut short any time-consuming discussions with patients, doctors claim that there are no significant studies in this field. Unfortunately, many patients rely on these views. There are however tons of scientific studies. Doctors simply cannot keep up with this important research. They do not even have time to keep up with the research in their own field. Medical knowledge doubles every three years. Lack of knowledge, time, and budget constraints are most often the reasons why doctors cut talks about vitamins and health short.

INFO

If you'd like to understand the importance of micronutrients in numerical terms, here are a few examples:
- In 129 studies, antioxidants reduced the risk of 13 types of cancer by 50%.
- Additional vitamin D and folate reduces the most commonly diagnosed types of cancers, which comprise more than 40% of all new cancer diagnoses. Vitamins E and C can reduce the risk of heart and circulatory system diseases by 30-40%.
- Supplemental folic acid could prevent 15,000 fatal heart and circulatory system diseases in Germany every year.
- High levels of folate in the blood significantly decrease the likelihood of developing dementia.
- The probability of developing cataracts can be reduced by 80%.
- Susceptibility to infections in winter can be decreased by 50%.

Thus, if you want to actively pursue the prevention of diseases with an improved diet and the additional benefits of micronutrients, you will have to get the information yourself. That is not an easy task. A lot of incorrect and poorly researched information is spread in the media. This is exactly why I have

> **TIP**
>
> Health starts at the molecular level, inside the 70 billion cells of your body. It's up to you to help every single one function optimally with the best possible supply of micronutrients, thereby preventing disease over the long term.

based my books on the research in large databases like the National Library of Medicine in Washington. Here I get all major studies in their original version. And it is worth looking at these studies and not just copying what some fellow journalist has written! I have chosen a vivid language, because science doesn't need to be boring and should be applicable to day-to-day life. It should lead to greater health and better performance. Study summaries give you a quick overview of current research that has direct consequences on how you can use nutrition to prevent cancer and other diseases. I have also inserted footnotes so the scientific sources can always be traced. Interviews with leading world experts show their perspective is on the topic. Many authors write about nutrition in a kind of religious way. You have to "believe" them. But, there is no research, footnotes or interviews with leading experts in their books. You often read speculation, individual opinions and generalisations of individual cases. You all know this from the latest diet crazes that are promoted every year. Most of them do not work in the long term. You may also know the poorly researched articles about vitamins that are nothing but confusing. I prefer to present you with the facts, the studies, the sources and the direct views of the researchers. You can build your own opinion based on the facts and develop strategies to pursue optimal health with these natural biocatalysts.

INFO

It sounds amazing, but, in the course of evolution, our immune system and metabolism developed on the basis of solely 47 vital, essential nutrients. These include 33 micronutrients - 13 vitamins, 6 minerals, and 14 trace elements. In addition, 2 fats (omega-6 and omega-3) and 8 amino acids are needed to make all protein structures. The body produces everything else it needs, but it is unable to do this without these substances. This makes the importance of an adequate supply of these micronutrients become quite clear.

Many governments already use this knowledge for cost savings in health care. They require that vitamins be added to certain basic staple foods. Folic acid is added to cereals, milk is required to have extra vitamin D, salt has added iodine and fertilizers are enriched with selenium so that selenium finds it way into the crops that we consume.

Nutrients are the basis of all life. They have proven themselves over millions of years as the best medicine, because during the course of evolution, the animals could not rely on a medical system and medications. Therefore a system "was developed" which repairs and regulates pathological changes of cells and changes in the genes. All these processes are dependent on an optimal supply of micronutrients. The billion of survival and metabolic trials and test over the cause of evolution (selection) have proven the essential need for these 47 micronutrients. No drug, with a few drug trials, can ever reach the potential that these nutrients have in the repair of your body. These tests were carried out "in real life" not in laboratories or with a couple of thousand patients. These nutrients function together as an alphabet – if one nutrient-letter is missing, then many metabolic words can only be put together fragmentarily. Micro-nutrients can penetrate into the nucleus of cells, where they have direct influence on the reading of gene sequences, and they activate and modulate the immune system. Therefore, a lack of these biocatalysts has a direct effect on metabolism and immune functions.

Living creatures with the best-functioning internal repair processes and most powerful immune system have a survival advantage. This fundamental law of nature holds true for humans, too, despite all the promises which high-tech medicine makes.

The short time it will take you to read this book will pay for itself in greater performance and in a longer, healthier life. And, for this you need the essential facts.

Andreas Jopp

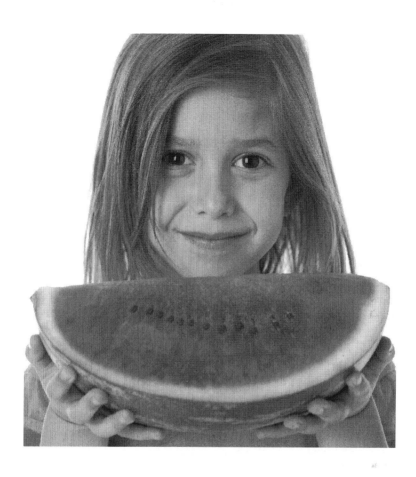

CHAPTER 1

How vitamins & minerals function

Would you fill your car with heating oil? Why can your biochemical factory only perform at its peak with the best biofuels? How do vitamins control your metabolism? Why do you only feel as good as your metabolism is working? How do antioxidants protect your 70 billion cells? Is there any way to detect cell damage at an early stage?

Your body as a biochemical factory

How do vitamins work, anyway?

Imagine for a moment… your own body as a giant biochemical factory: every second, billions of biochemical reactions are taking place in the 70 billion cells of your body. Vitamins, minerals, and trace elements accelerate all of these reactions – indeed, they couldn't happen without them. To produce a hormone, for example, or break down food, the metabolic processes run as though on a conveyor belt. They are divided into hundreds of individual biochemical steps, which take place in a strict order with the help of micronutrients.

Each individual cell of your body is a tiny factory of its own, with production facilities for protein molecules, power plants, trash incinerators, and copy machines for genetic information. Here, too, micronutrients are required for almost every step of the process. Your cells are a constant hive of biochemical activity, and never take a break. Accordingly, they need an uninterrupted supply of micronutrients. This is important, since many micronutrients can't be stored in the body – the vital, water-soluble B-vitamins, for example.

Why does vitamin deficiency slow the metabolism?

If a vitamin is missing at the start of a production process, the rest of the process can't continue, or can only take place through inefficient detours. The metabolism slows, and its efficiency decreases. Since the vitamins work together like a network, your metabolism is only as strong as the weakest link in this production chain.

A better metabolism with micronutrients

"Fuel up" with biofuels for your metabolic factory, instead of micronutrient-poor, worthless junk food. Most people understand that you shouldn't pour heating oil into the tank of a high-performance sports car, but they have lower standards when it comes to fueling their own bodies. What does your body really need? The answer is vitamins, minerals, and trace elements.

Today's athletes know how to make sure that these natural metabolic accelerants are present in their diets in sufficient quantities. That can even be measured: for every micronutrient, athletes often have blood levels in the upper third of the range. They benefit from this "micronutrient tuning". Pastured animals do the same thing, selecting the freshest and most vitamin-rich greens for grazing. You should also be getting the optimum quantity of micronutrients in your diet, since you're also working at peak performance,

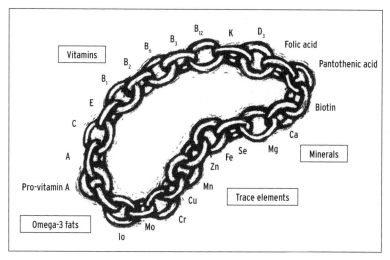

The metabolism is only as strong as its weakest link. Micronutrients work together.

both at home and on the job. Increase your mental and physical potential! Read the following information and learn something new about these biofuels. I promise you that the time you spend reading will pay for itself a hundred times over.

The importance of an optimal supply of micronutrients can be shown by the following examples:

- Vitamin C is used in 15,000 different metabolic processes. Whether hormone production or fat burning, it won't happen without the help of vitamin C.
- The eight B-complex vitamins play a role in all reactions of the energy metabolism, and regulate the nerve metabolism, including the brain and neurotransmitters (such as serotonin) which play an important role in your mood, motivation, and feeling of self-worth, but also in your memory, learning ability, and sleep quality. A deficiency of vitamin B may thus reveal itself in a lack of energy, difficulty concentrating, depression, and restlessness or even insomnia.
- The activity and effectiveness of the immune system in fighting against infections and tumors depends on an optimal supply of micronutrients. All immune cells need large quantities of such micronutrients in order to divide themselves and function.

INFO

If there is a shortage of any of the 47 essential micronutrients, your metabolism will slow down and your immune system will weaken. So, don't forget to refuel these biocatalysts regularly! You can reactivate many functions of your body's own biochemical factories, improve your performance, and support your immune system in preventing infections and other diseases.

Minerals and trace elements – building blocks of an active metabolism

Why do we need minerals and trace elements?

When you hear the words chromium, manganese, molybedenum, and zinc, most readers probably first think of car bumpers, or perhaps mineral deposits in the third world. However, these are precisely the substances that formed the building blocks of the first life forms. All the trace elements in our body wouldn't fill a teaspoon, yet human life would not exist without these inorganic elements.

Minerals and trace elements have several functions:
- They function as construction material for bones, for example calcium.
- They play a part in hundreds of metabolic reactions. For example, zinc is involved in the formation of more than 200 enzymes, and magnesium is important for more than 400. These enzymes manage our metabolism and our immune system.
- They bind heavy metals, enabling them to be excreted via our kidneys.
- They generate electrical impulses for the transmission of nerve impulses.
- They are an important component of hormones.
- They play a role in the "reading" and copying of genes.
- They perform a vital function in the immune system.
- They ensure that nutrients are pumped into and waste products out of the cells.
- They regulate the acid-base balance of the human body.

In many industrialized countries, there is a deficiency of zinc, chromium, iodine, and selenium in the food, as the soil has been depleted of these elements and the remnants of these vital trace elements found in the outer layers of grains are removed during processing. In such a state of deficiency, our metabolism is only functioning at a low rate. We can't escape our millennia-old genetic program.

Effective cell protection through antioxidant vitamins

How do vitamins protect your cells?

Vitamins also have another, completely different function, in addition to their metabolic importance. Certain vitamins – the antioxidants – protect your cells like a shield. Every single cell in your body is subjected to daily attacks by 10,000 free radicals! The cells would soon burst, if it weren't for the free radical-intercepting antioxidants such as vitamins A, C, and E that neutralize them before they can do harm. Trillions of free radicals are made harmless in just seconds.

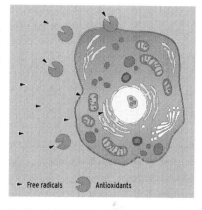

Free radicals   Antioxidants

Star Wars: Antioxidants intercept free radicals, thereby preventing them from penetrating the cells.

Forget Star Wars – you already possess the most incredible defense system that has ever been developed! However, since it's constantly in action, it also needs regular refueling.

You can see how that works in the illustration: antioxidants are intercepting free radicals to ensure that they never make it into the cells.

You can think of free radicals as something like single, incorrigible ladies' men: they're always trying to break electrons out of established electron bonds to bind their negative charge to themselves. Free radicals are oxidants, which means they steal electrons from other molecules and thus damage cells. In this way, within seconds, hundreds of thousands of electrons may change their "partner" – it's an orgy of free radicals!

Trace element protection – the body's own antioxidant enzymes

How do trace elements protect your cells?

If each cell is attacked 10,000 times a day by free radicals, and there are around 70 billion cells in the body, that makes some 7 trillion free radicals that need to be stopped every day. The antioxidant vitamins alone couldn't possibly handle this storm of free radicals; for that reason, the body produces its own potent antioxidant enzymes that "clean house" inside your body even more effectively than vitamins. These enzymes have a free electron, which they can transfer to free radicals in order to bind them harmlessly to themselves.

In order to produce this arsenal of natural enzymes, however, certain trace elements are necessary as raw materials. Without selenium, zinc, manganese, copper, and iron, which are all parts of enzyme complexes, production of these enzymes would fall short. The soil in many countries is especially poor in selenium and zinc. This is a consequence of the glacial period that washed these trace elements including iodine out of the soil. Of the other trace elements, up to 80% are lost during the extensive processing which grains are subjected to while being transformed into flour. That has significant negative consequences for our metabolism, since, without sufficient trace elements, not enough of the body's own antioxidant enzymes can be produced. The resulting failure to neutralize enough free radicals sets in motion the process of damage to the cells.

INFO

If there is a deficiency of antioxidant vitamins and of the multitude of plant-derived antioxidants, damage to the cells ensues, which results in the long term in cancer, cardiovascular disease, and other diseases caused by free radicals.

For this reason, all organisms attempt to neutralize free radicals with antioxidants. Plants that derive their energy from ultraviolet radiation protect their cells with more than 500 different antioxidants. These are often the plant pigments like the red lycopene in tomatoes. All living organisms are dependent on the supply of these plant-derived compounds for vitamins C and E, beta, lycopene and another 500 or so plant compounds also protect their organisms from free radicals.

Where are free radicals created?

Free radicals are created by numerous substances and processes:

- Everywhere that **energy** is produced in the cell, free radicals are generated as part of the normal metabolic processes.
- Everywhere that **oxygen** is being transported, free radicals can be found.
- Everywhere that **light (ultraviolet radiation)** reaches the body, free radicals are produced. This is why, for example, spending hours in the sun damages skin cells or the eyes. Free radicals attack the cells; this is why the eyes are especially well-protected with antioxidants.
- Certain **stress hormones** increase production of free radicals. Long-term stress can trigger free radical diseases such as cardiovascular disease and cancer.
- The **immune system** intentionally unleashes free radicals to destroy viruses and bacteria. If you develop an infection, such as of a viral influenza, the production of free radicals is boosted by the immune system – and, accordingly, the demand for antioxidants increased, since they have to intercept the excess free radicals once they've done their work of destroying the invading virus.
- Increasingly, we are also faced with **non-natural sources of free radicals**. These include environmental and household pollutants, many pharmaceuticals, synthetic drugs, and tobacco products. These free radical sources are increasingly responsible for cell damage and cancer.
- **X-rays** or other ionizing radiation absorbed on long-distance flights also produce free radicals.

In our modern world, these new sources of radicals can hardly be avoided. However, you now understand why a proper supply of antioxidants is becoming ever more important to neutralize free radicals and protect yourself. You certainly won't be able to accomplish this task with antioxidant-poor fast food.

The antioxidant network

The various antioxidants each neutralizes different free radicals. Vitamin E is fat-soluble, and is stored in the lipid-containing cell

> ### GOOD TO KNOW
>
> **Antioxidants - Cellular protectants**
> With the following protective substances (antioxidants), you can protect your cells against the destructive power of free radicals.
>
> - Vitamins: C, E
> - Vitaminoids: Coenzyme Q 10, alpha lipoic acid
> - Trace elements: selenium, zinc, manganese for antioxidant enzymes
> - Secondary plant compounds: Carotene (carrots), catechins (in green tea), lycopene (in tomatoes), polyphenols (red wine), flavonoids (citrus fruit), indoles (all types of cabbage), lutein (green leafy vegetables).

membranes to protect them. Vitamin C, by contrast, is water-soluble, and offers protection both in the cell and outside, in the watery environment of the blood. The plant-derived antioxidants are especially active in certain organs – lutein, for example, in the eyes. All oxidants cooperate with one another, as though in a network. For example, vitamin C takes on free radicals from vitamin E, thus "recycling" the rare and valuable vitamin E for reuse. The more dense a network you can build, with the widest variety of plant-derived antioxidants from fruit and vegetables, the better it will function. Thus, sound nutrition with lots of fruit and vegetables is the foundation for an adequate supply of the many plant-derived antioxidants – phytochemicals or secondary plant components. These plant-based antioxidants are mostly quite stable, so lycopene is still present in concentrated tomato paste.

The situation is quite different for the antioxidant vitamins and trace elements. After storage, transport, and processing, fruits and vegetables often contain only a fraction of their original micronutrients (see p. 93). That's always what most surprises some participants in my seminars. Despite the fact that many people pursue good nutrition, a micronutrient deficiency in 80% of the population is a sad fact, confirmed by study after study (see p. 80). It is thus ever more important to take in additional micronutrients as a supplement to your diet. That is how you can reach the level of vitamin and trace element intake on which our metabolism developed throughout evolution, back when everything was eaten fresh, uncooked, and unprocessed.

Only with a network of antioxidative compounds, as contained in fruits and vegetables, and supplementary micronutrients can the optimal protection against free radicals be reached today.

What damage do free radicals cause?

The damage caused to our cells by free radicals is enormous. Let's zoom into one of the cells in your body and see what free radicals do to it, and why healthy cells can mutate into cancerous ones.

You'll see the following symbols in the illustration on p. 22. They're meant to help you visualize what's happening.

 Free radicals start by attacking the cell membrane from the outside.

 Imagine the cell membrane as a busy port. Ships are constantly "docking" with the receptors and transporting raw materials (amino acids, lipids, micronutrients and energy) to the cell. Pumps and cranes are used to carry these vital substances from the outside to the interior of the cell.

✈   The cell membrane also has separate landing strips for information and orders (hormones) from the body, and extra landing strips for micronutrients.

💣   Free radicals bombard these port facilities and blast away fragments of these landing strips and transportation systems. The cell membranes lose the capacity to actively transport materials from outside into the cell, and to remove damaging substances (waste) from inside the cell. It shouldn't be hard to visualize the condition and functionality of your cells if they've been subjected to years of bombardment. Once free radicals have blown holes into your cell membranes, they can enter them more easily.

💾   Genetic material is especially affected by this process. It is your personal software, stored in the main control area of the cell nucleus, and contains all the important, saved instructions to control the entire cell. If your software "crashes" – even in part – various metabolic "programs" can no longer be read, or the metabolism is improperly regulated.

✂   Free radicals possess the capability to cut through proteins like a pair of scissors. They can slice through parts of cells and through DNA, the genetic code. Free radicals also affect communication between the cells.

💣   Free radicals destroy the tiny, water-filled channels through which the cells communicate with one another and ensure that no cell reproduces itself in an uncontrolled way, at the cost of other cells. If this communication channel is damaged, a malignant overgrowth of cells results. Thus, cancer is now considered to be one of the free radical diseases.

Another prime target for free radicals are the blood lipids. First, the attack of free radicals turns them "rancid" (oxidized), and then they tend to stick to the arterial walls by complex mechanisms. This much-feared clogging of the arteries is also called arteriosclerosis. Free radicals also attack the fat-containing sheath protecting the nerve and brain cells are involved in the development of Alzheimer's disease and dementia.

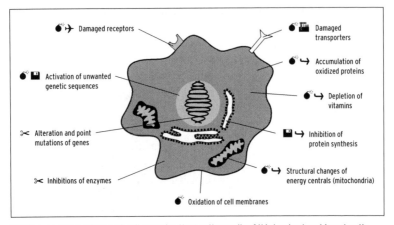

Damaged receptors

Damaged transporters

Accumulation of oxidized proteins

Activation of unwanted genetic sequences

Depletion of vitamins

Alteration and point mutations of genes

Inhibition of protein synthesis

Inhibitions of enzymes

Structural changes of energy centrals (mitochondria)

Oxidation of cell membranes

10,000 free radicals attack each cell every day. You see the results of this bombardment in and on the cell.

Free radicals also play a significant role in the aging process. Aging is an accumulation of changes in the software program that is your genetic code, which leads to changes in cells and a misguided metabolism. An ever-narrower transportation system is also part of growing older – each of us is only as old as his blood vessels. And aging also means the increasing decline of your nerve cells, expressed in reduced nerve conductivity and decreased mental functioning. The destructive effect of free radicals plays a role in all of these processes of aging.

Micronutrients - the real long-term insurance policy

What are free radical diseases?
Vitamins can help prevent unnecessary diseases, and thus save billions of dollars in health care costs. The results of major studies demonstrate that cardiovascular diseases, cancer, diabetes-induced vascular damage, and cataracts are often related to insufficient blood levels of antioxidants such as vitamin C, vitamin E, and plant-derived antioxidants. These diseases are known as free radical diseases. If sufficient quantities of antioxidants are available, these diseases are about 40% less likely to occur.

Mandatory enrichment with micronutrients
How important are these new studies for your own health? The medical studies on the extent of micronutrient deficiency and on the prevention of

disease are so convincing that various national governments now require by law that certain foods are fortified with micronutrients.

- Iodization of salt to prevent unnecessary thyroid surgeries
- Enrichment of milk with vitamin D to prevent osteoporosis
- Addition of selenium to fertilizers to prevent free radical diseases
- Addition of folic acid to basic foods in order to reduce embryonic malformations in pregnancy and reduce cardiovascular disease

In the long term, these governmental measures will pay off in several respects. As many countries have no such enrichment mandates, it is especially important to supplement these micronutrients yourself.

Prevention, rather than curing symptoms
In ancient China, a physician was paid for keeping his patients healthy. If one fell ill, he was treated free of charge. This focus on prevention in medicine has been lost over the centuries. Today, the emphasis is on the pharmaceutical treatment of diseases – or, more accurately, of symptoms – rather than on the maintenance of health. For good reason, nutrition and medicine were closely linked in ancient China. About 70% of our health care budget today is spent on treating the effects of nutritionally caused diseases.[1]

INFO

Vitamins are most helpful in preventing major diseases, rather than curing them. However, many people only pay attention to them once they've already developed health problems. Vitamins have both short-term and long-term effects.

Short-term:
- Improved performance.
- Powerful immune system.
- Reduction of symptoms resulting from vitamin deficiency.

Long-term:
Micronutrients are like an insurance policy for your health - the benefits aren't paid out until later. The earlier you start "paying in", the better this protective mechanism works. Among the "payouts" is cellular protection and a long-term reduction in the risk of certain age - related diseases:
- No. 1 Cause of death: heart and circulatory system diseases.
- No. 2 Cause of death: cancer.
- No. 1 Long-term care driver: dementia.
- No. 2 Long-term care driver: the osteoporosis avalanche.
- Protection against free radical damage to the eyes.

+++ SPECIAL: Getting enough vitamins? Measuring, not guessing +++

Cellular protection - do you get enough antioxidants?

Thanks to modern laboratory testing methods, it is now possible to measure whether cells have been damaged by a lack of antioxidants, and how badly. If perforated cell membranes or fragments of their DNA are found in your blood, it's a sure sign that your body's amazing defense system needs "refueling" with antioxidants more often. You need to do something about it: more fruits and vegetables and additional antioxidants such as vitamin C and selenium help to protect your cells. Try this antioxidant strategy for a few weeks, and then test your success. If your test results are in the clear, you've got the right mix of nutrition and antioxidants. Instead of discussing forever the pros and cons of vitamins and antioxidants, it's better to measure objectively – numbers say more than guesses. It's important to realize that precise antioxidant requirements may vary significantly from one person to another, depending on such factors as genes, lifestyle, exposure to damaging substances, or diseases. The test will let you know with certainty whether you're offering your cells the best protection possible. This varying need for vitamins is known as biochemical individuality.

How healthy are your cells?

The oxidative stress profile:

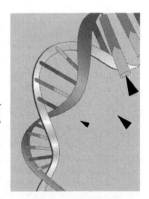

- The **PerOx test (lipid peroxidation)** tells us the extent to which the sensitive lipids in the cell membranes have already been attacked (oxidized) by free radicals.
- The **Deoxyguanosine test (OhdG test)** measures whether increasing quantities of DNA fragments, i.e. fragments of your cells' genetic software, are present in your blood. Once free radicals have penetrated the cellular membrane and made their way to the inside of the cell, parts of the cell's DNA software may be damaged. You can see this in the illustration.

Free radicals damage the body's DNA „software". Dissolved fragments of these genetic building blocks can be measured as oxidative damage.

How good is your antioxidative capacity?

The antioxidative capacity test shows whether your defensive systems against free radicals are working as they should be.

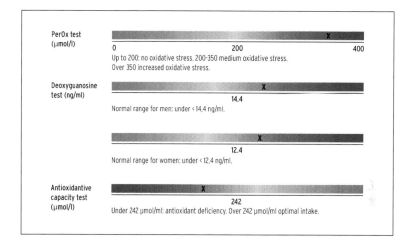

PerOx test (μmol/l)

0   200   400

Up to 200: no oxidative stress. 200-350 medium oxidative stress.
Over 350 increased oxidative stress.

Deoxyguanosine test (ng/ml)

14.4

Normal range for men: under < 14,4 ng/ml.

12.4

Normal range for women: under < 12,4 ng/ml.

Antioxidantive capacity test (μmol/l)

242

Under 242 μmol/ml: antioxidant deficiency. Over 242 μmol/ml optimal intake.

How to read the test

This oxidative stress profile shows the following results:

The "X" in the bar graph above corresponds to the value determined for the person tested.

For this patient, the **PerOx test** shows increased destruction of lipids in the cell membranes.

The **deoxyguanosine test** also shows elevated levels, and indicates that damage to the patient's DNA is occurring at an elevated rate.

The patient's **antioxidative capacity** is at a low level. The reason for the cellular damage thus appears to be an undersupply of antioxidants.

Who can measure potential cell damage and my own antioxidant requirements?

Free radicals damage the body's DNA "software". Dissolved fragments of these genetic building blocks can be measured as oxidative damage.

There are specialised medical laboratories performing these types of tests. Consult your doctor to have a blood sample drawn, and ask that he submits it to one of these labs. The quality of the laboratory is crucial for ensuring the reliability of the results.

25

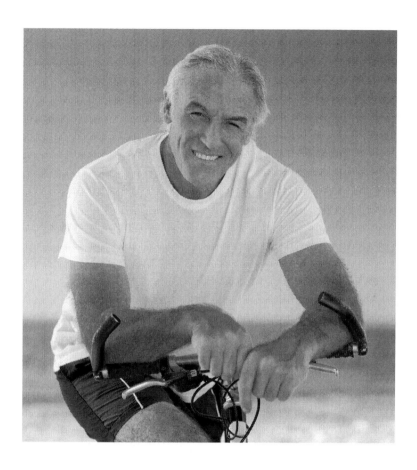

CHAPTER 2

Vitamins – your insurance policy

Why do Vitamin C and E reduce heart and cardio-vascular diseases? Why does B-vitamin deficiency double the risk of such diseases? How do extra Vitamin D and Folic acid help prevent the most common cancers? How do antioxidants protect the brain? Why do B-vitamins reduce the risk of dementia? How does one build a strong skeletal structure and avoid osteoporosis? How do antioxidants help protect your eyes?

Cardiovascular disease - most common cause of death

Cardiovascular disease causes 45% of all deaths in the Western world – more than any other. Every second citizen in the developed world dies of cardiovascular disease.

Through the consumption of additional micronutrients, this risk can be cut in half. Presumably, some readers are thinking:

"That kind of prevention is just too easy, and too cheap."

With that thought, you're hitting on a key problem of the health care industry: vitamins are cheap, and non-patentable. Expensive regulatory approval procedures for vitamins as prescription drugs are thus not remotely worthwhile for the pharmaceutical industry. However, since drug regulatory laws only permit drugs with regulatory approval to make medical claims on their packaging, you will never see any such medical information on a package of vitamins for legal reasons.

> ### GOOD TO KNOW
>
> **Risk Factors**
> Vitamin deficiency plays a major role in the development of cardiovascular (heart and circulatory system) diseases:
> - Risk factor 1: clogged arteries resulting from oxidized blood lipids, as the blood contains too little vitamin C, vitamin E, selenium, and other plant-based antioxidants.
> - Risk factor 2: high blood levels of homocysteine, due to inadequate metabolization of homocysteine as a consequence of low levels of vitamin B_6, folate/folic acid, and vitamin B_{12}.

"But my doctor never told me about this!"

The most interesting studies were conducted around the mid-1990s. It takes about 20 years until scientific results make their way into practice – if they ever do at all. Out of every 100 scientific discoveries, only about five ever appear in the medical practice, 20 years later. That was demonstrated by a 21-million-Euro research program carried out by the German Ministry of Health and the German health insurance industry.[2]

"My doctor told me: 'there are no studies proving that.'"

Vitamins play almost no role in medical research studies. Most doctors know only that we need sufficient vitamins. Furthermore, doctors aren't paid for patients' avoidance of diseases, but for curing symptoms of diseases with medication. To help you counter this "nobody's shown that…"-prejudice, you'll find numerous short tables in this chapter presenting the most important studies that you should know about to maintain your own health.

Antioxidant deficiencies and cardiovascular diseases

In the 1980s, it was still thought that high levels of cholesterol in the blood were the main risk factor for cardiovascular diseases. Today, we know that cholesterol only clogs the arteries once it is oxidized by free radicals – when it goes rancid, so to speak – due to insufficient levels of antioxidants such as Vitamin C and E in the blood.

So how does that work exactly? Visualize for a moment your 240,000 km of blood vessels, through which blood lipids are constantly being pumped. Each one of these lipid particles contains, among other things, 1,400 fat molecules, which can all too easily be oxidized by free radicals and stick to the arterial wall. To prevent this, five to nine molecules of vitamin E ride along on every blood lipid particle and intercept the free radicals. Your vitamin E intake determines how many of these helpful, free-radical-catching molecules of vitamin E are in your blood. Six studies have shown that, the higher a person's vitamin E intake, the fewer blood lipids can be oxidized.[3]

Many large population studies point to the same conclusion. Blood levels of vitamin E are a better predictor of future heart attacks than cholesterol levels.[4] High levels of cholesterol were linked with heart attacks in 29% of cases, while low levels of vitamin E were predictive in 70% of cases![5]

Low vitamin levels - high heart attack risk

Why do you need more vitamin E with high blood lipid levels?
The two risk factors for cardiovascular diseases – high blood lipid levels and low levels of vitamin E – are closely related. Two-thirds of all Germans have elevated lipid levels as a consequence of being overweight and consuming a high-fat diet. Today, more blood lipids are being carried through the body's blood vessels than ever before in human evolutionary history. The more lipids

being circulated, the greater the risk that these fats become oxidized. Due to our increased intake of dietary fat, you need more vitamin E than ever before to safeguard these little shipments of fat in your blood.

The MONICA study carried out by the World Health Organization (WHO), which gathered information in 16 European countries, confirms: in 87% of all cases, a correlation could be established between heart attack risk and insufficient levels of vitamin C and E in the bloodstream. You already know about the function of vitamin C: it restores vitamin E by taking on the free radicals it has absorbed.

40 to 100% of the population does not even get the minimum daily recommended amount of vitamin E – 12 mg per day – through dietary intake. For this reason, many scientists recommend additional low dosed (up to 200mg) vitamin E per day for optimal prevention of diseases of the heart and circulatory system.

Antioxidants reduce heart and circulatory system diseases

Each year, 274,000 Germans suffer a heart attack. In terms of air travel, that would be like three plane crashes every day. With odds like that, no-one would be willing to board a plane without a parachute, to say nothing of other safety measures. When it comes to heart and circulatory system diseases, though, few people think about such precautions. With adequate vitamin E alone, the risk of a "crash", i.e. a heart attack, could be reduced by around 40%.

Two Harvard University studies carried out over the course of eight years on 87,000 nurses[6] and 40,000 doctors[7] showed that the risk of cardiovascular diseases could be reduced by 41% by a daily consumption of 100 to 200 mg of vitamin E. A daily intake of 200 mg of vitamin E showed the best results, with a reduction in mortality of approximately 34%.

High dosed vitamin E on the other hand proved to be counter productive. While low dose studies show beneficial effects, high dose studies are inconclusive. The message here: more is not always better. Supplementing is something different than flooding your system with vitamin E. Vitamin E is a fat-soluble vitamin like vitamin A and vitamin D. Fat-soluble vitamins should not be overdosed.

Has your doctor ever measured your vitamin E level?

If you suffer from cardiovascular disease or high blood lipids, your doctor should measure your vitamin E levels. Has your doctor even recommended vitamin E to you? Incidentally, many cardiologists (heart doctors) themselves take vitamin E. In a study of 181 leading American cardiologists, 39% took vitamin E![8]

How vitamin E reduces the risk of cardiovascular diseases

The clearest evidence for the risk-reducing effect of vitamin E on cardiovascular diseases comes from long-term studies on patients who were all healthy at the start of the study. Vitamin E's effect is primarily preventive, reducing the likelihood of developing cardiovascular diseases. Whether and how vitamin E reduces mortality among patients with existing cardiovascular disease is still being studied. Some studies involving such patients show no positive effect, while others, such as one carried out by the University of Cambridge, point to a reduction of 70% in the probability of suffering a second heart attack.[9] Further studies are continuing on this topic.

Someone told you vitamin E had „no effect"?

It's important to realize that, when you hear about studies in which vitamin E did not reduce the risk of developing heart and circulatory system diseases, those studies were most likely ones involving people who had already developed such diseases – in other words, studies of the therapeutic effects of vitamin E. Since the popular press and even some doctors don't clearly distinguish between studies of prevention and those of therapeutic treatments, certain muddled preconceived notions about vitamins have spread. Vitamins are primarily important in preventing diseases from occurring, in other words for avoiding damage in the first place – and vitamin E is crucial here.

How does vitamin E work?

It functions not only as an antioxidant (protecting blood lipids from oxidation), but works on many other levels in preventing cardiovascular diseases:

- Vitamin E makes the blood platelets less sticky, so they're less likely to attach themselves to the arterial wall.
- Vitamin E makes the blood less viscous, so it flows more easily through narrowed blood vessels.
- Vitamin E reduces the blood's ability to clot, much like aspirin. It extends the time in which you bleed before a clot closes the wound. That's very important with partially clogged, narrowed arteries, as vitamin E reduces the likelihood that a clot in a narrowed artery blocks the blood flow to the heart or brain. These clots are the cause of two-thirds of all heart attacks and strokes.
- Vitamin E, like aspirin, reduces inflammation factors. Men with a high level of inflammatory messengers suffer heart attacks at three times the rate of men with lower levels – and this risk is completely independent of blood lipid levels.[10] It's long been understood that only half of all heart

attack patients have elevated lipid levels! It is becoming more and more clear that one of the main causes for changes to the blood vessels is an inflammatory process. Vitamin E plays a positive role in this context.

Vitamin E & Omega-3: how they work

- Omega-3 fatty acid works primarily on the inflammatory messengers. In conjunction with additional omega-3 lipids from fish, vitamin E has the greatest effect in reducing the risk of developing cardiovascular diseases. Fats aren't the focus of this book, but you can learn more about undertaking your own, vital "oil change", with fewer killer fats and more healthy ones. This "oil change" can cut heart and circulatory system disease in half. Here, too, vitamin E plus omega-3 fatty acid is an unbeatable combination. Vitamin E lowers risk by another 20% in comparison with omega-3 alone.

Professor Lauterbach of the University of Cologne's Institute for Health Economics has calculated that vitamin E could help the German health care system save 4.6 billion euros per year.

Why do we need more vitamin E?

For about the past hundred years, we have been eating twice as much fat as in the previous two million years of human history. Our metabolism hasn't yet adapted to this. A good 30–35% of our daily caloric intake comes from sticky fats, which flood the arteries after a hearty meal. To transport this load of lipids through the bloodstream in safety, you need much more vitamin E to protect them from free radicals.

How much vitamin E is actually needed?

Vitamin E metabolites are found in urine.[17] These products of vitamin E metabolization appear with a daily intake of roughly 100 mg of vitamin E. That's about five times the daily recommended allowance in Germany – certainly food for thought! In other words, only at an intake above 100 mg does the body recognize there to be an excess of vitamin E and get rid of it – but then only some of it. Some is stored in the eyes, in the cell membranes, and on the blood lipids as a protection against free radicals.

Which is the best vitamin E?

Artificial vitamin E is only half as effective as the natural kind. That means that 200 mg of artificial vitamin E have the same effect as 100 mg of natural vitamin E. Read the information on the package: natural vitamin E is d-alpha-tocopherol, while artificial is dl-alpha-tocopherol.

Studies: Vitamin E lowers the risk of cardiovascular diseases

Participants	Period	Results
87,245 women	10 years	↓ **41%** lower risk of fatal cardiovascular diseases compared with participants not taking vitamin E.[11]
39,910 men	4 years	↓ **32%** lower risk of fatal cardiovascular diseases compared with participants not taking vitamin E.[12]
5,133 women and men	12 years	↓ **32%** lower risk of fatal cardiovascular diseases.[13]
11,178 women and men	8 years	↓ **41%** lower risk of fatal cardiovascular diseases.[14]
Omega-3 fatty acids reduce cardiovascular diseases		
76,000 women	10 years	↓ **43%** lower risk of fatal heart attacks with high consumption of omega-3 fats.[15]
Vitamin E + omega-3: An unbeatable combination		
76,000 women	10 years	↓ **64%** lower risk of fatal heart attacks with high consumption of omega-3 fats and supplemental vitamin E.[16]

How do I take vitamin E?

Always with food, and never on an empty stomach, since vitamin E is fat-soluble and a much larger percentage of the vitamin is absorbed into the bloodstream in this manner.

Vitamin C reduces the chances for cardiovascular-diseases

This is how it works:
- It intercepts free radicals and thus protects blood lipids from oxidation.
- It takes on free radicals from other antioxidants, thus recycling the antioxidants for further free radical-scavenging.
- By reducing the number of free radicals, fewer inflammatory messengers are produced. These messengers are a primary cause of heart and circulatory system diseases.
- Vitamin C restores the functionality of the arterial wall, helping it to widen under higher pressure and thus avoid developing tiny but dangerous cracks.
- In addition, vitamin C helps reduce the formation of fatty deposits on the arterial walls.

Studies: Vitamin C reduces the risk of cardiovascular diseases

Participants	Period	Results
85,118 women	16 years	↓ **28%** lower risk of cardiovascular diseases among participants consuming supplemental vitamin C. Vitamin C-rich dietary intake alone did not lead to a reduction in risk.[18]
11,348 men and women	10 years	↓ **25%** lower risk of cardiovascular diseases among women and Ð42 % lower among men who attained an intake level of at least 300 mg per day through dietary intake and supplemental vitamin C.[19]
292,172 men and women	analysis of 9 studies	↓ **25%** lower risk of cardiovascular diseases among participants consuming more than 700 mg of supplemental vitamin C.[20]
2,000 men and women	20 years	↓ **29%** lower risk of stroke among participants with the highest blood levels of vitamin C in comparison with the participants with the lowest levels.[21]
2,773 men and women	–	↓ **33%** lower risk of coronary artery among participants with the highest blood levels of vitamin C in comparison with the participants with the lowest levels.[22]

How do studies work?

Wouldn't it be interesting to observe healthy people and find out what diseases they develop based on how they eat? That's exactly what the Harvard studies do. For 20 years, these studies have been recording the health of 167,000 people, all of whom were in good health at the start of the studies, without cardiovascular diseases, cancer, or diabetes. 116,000 nurses and 51,500 doctors are participating in the studies. Their nutritional behavior and other information are collected regularly. Nurses and doctors were chosen because they can most reliably report medical diagnoses and changes to their health. These are among the largest observational studies of their kind. Six professors at Harvard University and some two dozen statisticians, doctors, and graduate students are busy running the study and examining its results.

How do scientists know that it is vitamin C that reduces cardiovascular diseases, and not some other nutrient? The studies and databases are so immense that a group such as "people with similar vitamin C intake" can be divided into many subgroups, depending on what else they eat and what other risk factors they have. In this way, the various vitamins and other nutrients can be analyzed separately for clues about their effects. It is also possible to analyze precisely various risk factors in the subgroups, such as smoking, obesity, and a lack of exercise, to determine whether these affect the results. From these evaluations, it is known that the reduction in cardiovascular disease risk caused by vitamin C is a valid result, as all risk factors and other nutrients have been accounted for in the analysis. Smaller studies are unable to do this, as their numbers are simply not statistically significant enough. You'll "meet" the doctors and nurses of this study several more times while making your way through this book.

> **TIP**
>
> Some interesting information: in these studies, a diet rich in vitamin C by itself did little to reduce the risk of cardiovascular diseases. Only a higher vitamin C intake with vitamin supplements lowered the risk by about 25%. The reason: only with a daily intake of 400 mg of vitamin C are the cells optimally provisioned with vitamin C for intercepting free radicals.[23] Only with an intake of at least 500 mg do the studies demonstrate the restoration of the production of nitrite oxide, which is responsible for the flexibility of the arterial walls. Vitamin C has no undesirable side effects and can safely be taken in high doses.

Selenium deficiency and cardiovascular diseases

In addition to vitamins C and E from external sources, the body produces its own antioxidant enzymes to neutralize free radicals. One of the primary components of these enzymes is the trace element selenium, which protects blood lipids against going "rancid" and keeps the heart muscle stable.

It is interesting to compare the blood levels of selenium in heart attack patients with those who have not had heart attacks: such comparisons are called case control studies. In 11 such studies, a reduction of 57% in cardiovascular disease risk was shown.[24] Even if the selenium studies aren't conclusive, the protection against free radicals by this trace element points in the same direction. It's worth noting that the studies in which a severe selenium deficiency was eliminated showed the clearest results.

Folate reduces homocysteine

Have you ever had your homocysteine levels measured?

No? Have you even heard of this term before? Many doctors still do not regularly perform this test, even though homocysteine is one of the most important risk factors for cardiovascluar diseases. Tragically, according to a study carried out by the University of Bonn, only 5% of internal medicine doctors even knew what homocysteine was, and that it can be reduced by certain B-vitamins. People with high homocysteine levels have a risk of a heart attack three times as high as those with normal levels. The risk of a stroke is increased by a factor of four.

Dangerous homocysteine levels

Ideally, your homocysteine levels should be under 10 μmol/L. Higher values usually point to a B-vitamin deficiency. Without the presence of folate, vitamin B_6, and vitamin B_{12}, homocysteine cannot be metabolized. This causes homocysteine levels to rise, and promotes the formation of plaques in the arteries. Interestingly, then, a homocysteine test also provides the best information as to whether you're getting enough B-vitamins. If the value is too high, it shows that for your genetic or individual needs your intake of B-vitamins is not adequate. With the objective measures of homocysteine, you can shorten the pro and con debate about vitamins.

Things are often very different if you measure actual blood levels of the B-vitamins. You'll often be told that your values are "within the normal range" – but what range is that? To set the average values of poorly-nourished people as the recommended norm is a very poor criterion. Homocysteine levels thus often provide better information about whether you're getting enough B-vitamins.

Incidentally, supplemental vitamin B_6, folic acid, and vitamin B_{12} can reduce homocysteine levels by about 30%. This has been shown in more than 25 different studies.[25] This corresponds to a drastically lower heart attack risk. About 80% of men and 90% of women don't get their minimum daily recommended dose of folate! About 50% to 90% don't take in enough vitamin B6. People older than 70 almost always show a deficiency of vitamin B_{12}, as they are less able to absorb it than younger people. For this reason, the risk of stroke in older people drops by 21% when high doses of vitamin B_{12} are consumed.[26, 27]

Vitamin pills reduce the risk of cardiovascular diseases better

Let's go back to those 80,000 nurses from the Harvard study mentioned above. The nurses with the highest intake of vitamin B_6 and folate / folic acid (i.e., folate from food and folic acid from supplements) suffered 45% fewer heart attacks over 14

> **TIP**
>
> Folic acid is heat-stable and is thus used in vitamin products and in foods as an additive in place of folate. You should consume 400 mcg of supplementary folic acid every day. Important: always look closely at the composition of multivitamins. Some multivitamins contain little or no folic acid.

years.[28] It's important to know that folate is the most sensitive of all vitamins. 90% is lost in storage and cooking. For this reason, the scientists conducting the study examined whether participants using multivitamins with folic acid (which is heat-insensitive and storable) did better on average than those who met their folate intake through diet alone. The results: the nurses who used multivitamins had a risk reduction 25% greater than that of the participants who relied on fruits and vegetables alone.

Studies: Additional folate reduces the risk of cardiovascular diseases and strokes and lowers blood pressure

Participants	Period	Results
70,082 women	14 years	↓ **45%** lower risk of cardiovascular diseases among women with the highest combined folate/folic acid intake from diet and supplementation together[29]
43,732 men	14 years	↓ **29%** lower risk of stroke caused by inadequate blood flow with the highest intake of folate/folic acid[30]
Meta-analysis of 8 studies	–	↓ **18%** lower risk of stroke through additional folic acid supplementation ↓ **28%** lower risk of stroke with folic acid supplementation lasting longer than three years[31]
1,015 men	10 years	**Folate blood values** ↓ **65%** lower risk of stroke in men with the highest folate blood levels[32]
93,803 younger women (27-44 years) 62,260 older women (43-70 years)	8 years	**Folic acid and blood pressure** With 800 mcg of supplementary folic acid: ↓ **45%** lower risk of high blood pressure among younger women ↓ **39%** lower risk of high blood pressure among older women[33]
2,155 men and women over 66 years	11 years	**Older people and supplementary vitamin B_{12}** ↓ **21%** lower risk of stroke and cardiovascular diseases with high-dose intake of vitamin B_{12}[34]

Even more reliable than surveys of vitamin intake are measurements of folate levels in the blood. High blood levels of folate correspond with a 65% reduction in the likelihood of strokes.

It's recently been discovered that high folate intake via vitamin tablets (800 mcg) also reduces the risk of high blood pressure, which is the cause of 50% of heart attacks and 70% of strokes. These levels are simply unattainable through a healthy diet alone. Folic acid is a clear example of how vitamin supplementation provides a noticeable reduction in risk when compared with a healthy, balanced diet alone.

So, why all these studies? Well, next time your doctor tells you that there are no studies on this or that topic, you'll know better.

> **GOOD TO KNOW**
>
> **Effective substances against cardio-vascular diseases**
> Vitamins C and E and selenium prevent the oxidation of blood lipids. Vitamins C and E fight cardiovascular disease in other ways, too. Folic acid, vitamin B6 (and, for older people, also vitamin B12) lower homocysteine levels. Started early enough, supplementing with additional micronutrients helps sharply lower the risk of cardiovascular diseases.

It has been calculated that, in the United States, 56,000 deaths from cardiovascular diseases could be prevented every year by correcting folate deficiencies. Professor Pietrzik of the University of Bonn estimates the number of avoidable deaths for Germany at 15,000 per year.

Since 1998, United States law has required that all grain products be enriched with folic acid in order to compensate for the folate deficiency. It's a measure that costs almost nothing, but helps save billions of dollars in subsequent health costs.

Potassium & magnesium against high blood pressure

In every sense, we live our lives under pressure. 31% of Americans have high blood pressure. High blood pressure was listed as a primary or contributing cause of death for 326,000 Americans. In 2010, high blood pressure will cost the United States $76.6 billion in health care services, medications, and missed days of work. High blood pressure is the main cause behind 50% of all heart attacks and 70% of all strokes. 45% of deaths of people over the age of 65 can be blamed on high blood pressure. 30% of patients with high blood pressure don't even know that they're subjecting their heart and blood vessels to excessive pressure, and don't know about the damage that results. Imagine driving with tires over - filled with air over a road with a hundred thousand potholes, day in and day out. But of course you'd never do that. Well, that's what high blood pressure does to your heart. Its primary cause is excessive weight; weight loss immediately lowers blood pressure.

It's amazing – studies show that potassium and magnesium can lower blood pressure regardless of any weight loss. The risk of cardiovascular diseases and strokes drops with the consumption of potassium-rich fruits and vegetables by approximately 30–40 %. Innumerable studies have confirmed the successful use of magnesium in preventing cardiovascular diseases such as acute myocardial infarction, heart rhythm disturbances, angina pectoris, cardiac muscle weakness, heart valve problems, and strokes. And we see the familiar phenomenon: magnesium is not patentable, and costs pennies in comparison to the various pharmaceutical products.

Fruits & vegetables against cardiovascular diseases

Studies: Fruits and vegetables lower the risk of cardiovascular diseases and strokes

Participants	Period	Results
Meta-analysis of 11 studies of 278,459 men and women	11 years (average of all studies)	↓ **27%** lower risk of cardiovascular diseases among participants who regularly ate 5 portions of fruits and vegetables daily rather than 3.[37]
Meta-analysis of 8 studies of 257,551 men and women	13 years (average of all studies)	↓ **26%** lower risk of stroke among participants who regularly ate 5 portions of fruits and vegetables daily rather than 3 portions.[38]
75,596 women and 38,683 men	14 years and 8 years	↓ **31%** lower risk of stroke among participants with the highest intake of fruits and vegetables. Each additional daily portion reduces the risk by 6%.[39]
84,251 women and 42,148 men	14 years and 8 years	↓ **20%** lower risk of cardiovascular diseases among participants with the highest intake of fruits and vegetables. Each additional daily portion reduces the risk by 4%.[40]

Additional intake of vitamin C (400 mg), vitamin E (100 mg), and folic acid (400 mcg) showed a statistically independent reduction in risk, even in people who ate diets rich in fruits and vegetables. The reason for this is likely that these high dosages cannot be achieved through diet alone. So, vitamin supplements help – but supplements are no excuse for poor nutrition! Vitamins aren't a substitute, but an extra support in the network of antioxidants. Fruits and vegetables reduce the risk of cardiovascular diseases by about 30%: plant-derived antioxidants prevent the oxidation of blood lipids, B-vitamins lower homocysteine, fiber reduces blood lipid levels, and potassium and magnesium lower dangerous high blood pressure levels and thus the risk of strokes and heart attacks. In the Harvard studies, green leafy vegetables and broccoli (in other words, vegetables with high folate content) and citrus fruit (i.e. fruits rich in Vitamin C) performed best.[35, 36] It was precisely these vitamins that caused the greatest reduction in risk in the vitamin studies. Every additional daily portion of fruits and vegetables lowers the risk of cardiovascular diseases and strokes by 5-6%. So eat as many fruits and vegetables as you can, but at least five portions a day.

Cancer - second most common cause of death

It's frightening to realize that more than 400,000 new cases of cancer are diagnosed in Germany each year. Looking at the distribution of cancer deaths by age, one notices that people are being afflicted at ever younger ages, and that the prevalence of cancer is increasing. Is it just fate that affects our likelihood of developing cancer? Or, are we paying for our failure to take adequate precautions? What would you give if you knew that you could reduce that risk by 50%? You may think this is an exaggeration, but research results point in this direction.

Antioxidants reduce the frequency of cancer

In a comprehensive meta-study, Professor Block of the University of California at Berkeley evaluated 164 medical studies examining 13 different types of cancer. In 129 studies, it was shown that the average cancer rate was lowered by 50% if a high supplemental intake of antioxidants (vitamin C, vitamin E, and plant-based antioxidants) was consumed daily. The preventive role of additional antioxidant vitamins and plant-derived antioxidants found in fruits and vegetables is now undisputed in the scientific world for certain types of cancer.

The National Cancer Research Institute in the United States evaluated 47 clinical studies to examine the effect of vitamin C.[42] 34 of these studies showed that the participants with the highest measured amounts of vitamin C in their blood decreased their cancer risk by half.

The mechanism is always the same: antioxidants defend cells and their genetic information from damage, preventing them from degenerating. Certain antioxidants

> **TIP**
>
> The National Cancer Institute (NCI) discussed a daily consumption of at least 225 mg of vitamin C, unless there are additional stressors present, such as smoking or diabetes. That's almost three times the amount recommended by German authorities.[41]

40

can also bind heavy metals and other pollutants and permit them to be excreted from the body.

Many studies have shown a direct link between raised vitamin C levels in the blood and a lowered cancer risk:

Cancer type	Number of studies	Direct positive correlation (statistically significant)
Esophagus, mouth, trachea	8	8
Stomach	6	6
Lung	9	5
Pancreas	6	4
Intestine	8	4
Uterus	5	4
Colon	5	3
Total	47	34

Vitamins lower the frequency of cancer

Nature has assigned the vitamins several million functions in the metabolic process. Scientists don't fully understand all of them, yet. However, it is noticeable that precisely those vitamins of which we have the greatest deficiencies – folate, vitamin B6, and vitamin D – are also the most effective in lowering the risk of certain cancers. Just correcting this deficiency already drastically lowers the chances of cancer.

Vitamin D deficiency

90% of Germans don't get enough vitamin D. Vitamin D is created by the effect of sunlight on the skin; however, in these northern latitudes, there isn't get much sun during the winter months. Is there a geographical distribution of cancer cases? Certain scientists noticed that the prevalence of cancer – excluding skin cancer– was higher in the northern states of the U.S.A., which get relatively little sun, than it was in the southern states.[43] Add to this that evolution did not intend for humans to be creatures that live by artificial light, yet we spend most of our time indoors. Our entire metabolism was, and is, designed for a high and constant production of vitamin D through a life spent outdoors. Vitamin D regulates many hormone-induced processes, and has an influence on the immune system, which destroys cancer cells; prevents their cell division and promotes apoptosis – the self-destruction program of cancer cells. So, it should come as no surprise that a vitamin D deficiency plays a major role in the development of cancer. There's no question that it pays to address this deficiency.

Vitamin D reduces the risk of the most common types of cancer

Vitamins don't have the same preventive effect on all types of cancer. It is interesting, however, that vitamin D is effective for precisely the most commonly found kinds of cancer. Prostate and intestinal cancers are the cause of 39% of all new cancer diagnoses amongst men, while breast and intestinal cancers are responsible for 44% of all new cancer cases amongst women.

B-vitamin deficiencies and the most common cancers

There are several other substances of which we tend to have a deficiency, and which have an effect on new cancer diagnoses. 90% of all Germans don't get enough folic acid, and 60–70% need more vitamin B_6. The B-vitamins are particularly important in the crucial task of repairing damaged DNA, in other words fixing the cell's genetic code. Is it really surprising that correcting this deficiency has a drastic effect on the risk of developing various cancers? If you still believe that additional vitamins "don't accomplish much", I'd like to try one final time to convince you otherwise by underscoring the following numbers: folate and vitamin B_6 reduce the risk of breast, ovarian, and intestinal cancers, which together are responsible for 50% of all new cancer diagnoses in women. In men, these vitamins reduce the likelihood of developing intestinal, prostate, and probably lung cancers, which are the causes of 53% of all new cancer diagnoses among men.

The importance of B-vitamins is especially clear among men and women who regularly drink alcohol. In the studies, even small amounts of alcohol – 15 g per day, about 1 to 2 glasses of wine – have a sharply negative effect. Alcohol drastically reduces vitamin B_6 and folate levels, thus increasing the risk of cancer. Just avoiding this B-vitamin deficiency brings a significant improvement in risk profile. For example, the highest blood levels of folate reduce the likelihood of developing breast cancer by 27% in women. For women who drink alcohol every day, the risk is reduced by 90%. The story is much the same for ovarian cancer: high doses of folate lower the risk by 33%, and by 74% among women who are daily drinkers (see also p. 44).

INFO

Vitamins aren't "alternative medicine"; they work in a scientifically provable manner and are thus a part of academic medicine. No pension scheme can reward you so well as investing in your vitamin intake.

Studies: Vitamin D against common cancers

Participants	Period	Results
47,800 men	14 years	↓ **29%** lower risk of death from cancer with high vitamin D blood levels ↓ **45%** lower risk of developing cancers of the digestive system[44]
14,916 men	18 years	↑ Doubled risk of prostate cancer with low vitamin D blood levels[45]
46,771 men and 75,427 women	14 years 16 years	↓ **41%** lower risk of pancreatic cancer in populations with high vitamin D blood levels in comparison with those having low vitamin D blood levels[46]
Meta-analysis of 5 studies	-	↓ **49%** lower risk of intestinal cancer with high a vitamin D intake[47]
19,000 men	13 years	↑ Risk of prostate cancer three times as high in men with low blood levels of vitamin D in their blood[48]
88,691 women	16 years	↓ **28%** lower risk of breast cancer with high vitamin D intake[49]

Multivitamins for optimal protection

Let's not fool ourselves: it's an almost impossible task. In our modern, high-stress world, in which home and work are ever farther apart and we eat away from home ever more often, how are we supposed to reach even the minimal necessary intake of folate and vitamin B_6? In order to prevent cardiovascular diseases and cancer, we should definitely aim for a better higher intake and blood levels of these micronutrients. Given the significant vitamin losses resulting from storage and processing of foods, we just can't rely on a few leaves of lettuce on the edge of our plates. You should definitely supplement your supply of these delicate vitamins with a good multivitamin product. Compare how much you pay each month for health insurance with how little it would cost to insure your health with vitamins!

Studies: Folate and vitamin B$_6$

Participants	Period	Results
Folic acid and Vitamin B$_6$ against breast and ovarian cancer		
32,826 women	13 years	↓ **27%** lower risk of breast cancer among women with the highest levels of folate in their blood ↓ **90%** lower risk of breast cancer among women who drink alcohol daily, but have the highest levels of folate in their blood[51]
32,826 women	13 years	↓ **30%** lower risk of breast cancer among women with the highest levels of vitamin B$_6$ in the blood[52]
62,739 post-menopausal women	9 years	↓ **22%** lower risk of breast cancer among women with the highest folate intake[53]
88,818 women	16 years	↓ **45%** lower risk of breast cancer among women with the highest folate intake[54]
34,387 post-menopausal women	12 years	↑ **21%** higher risk of breast cancer among women with low folate intake[55]
Case control study of 2,703 women with breast cancer compared with women without breast cancer	–	↓ **27%** lower risk of breast cancer among women with the highest folate intake[56]
61,084 women	13 years	↓ **27%** lower risk of ovarian cancer among women with the highest folate intake ↓ **74%** lower risk of ovarian cancer among women who drink alcohol daily and have the highest folate intake[57]
Folic acid against prostate cancer and lung cancer		
65,836 men	9 years	↓ **22%** lower risk of prostate cancer among men with the highest folate intake[58]
Case control study of 2,745 men with prostate cancer compared with men without prostate cancer	–	↓ **34%** lower risk of prostate cancer among men with the highest folate intake ↓ **54%** lower risk of prostate cancer among men with the lowest alcohol intake and highest folate intake[59]
58,279 men	6 years	↓ **37%** lower risk of lung cancer among smokers with the highest folate intake[60]

Participants	Period	Results
Folate and vitamin B$_6$ against intestinal cancer		
88,758 women[6]	16 years	↓ **20%** lower risk of intestinal cancer among women with 400mcg of supplemental folate intake ↓ **51%** lower risk of intestinal cancer among women with a higher genetically-caused risk with 400 mcg of supplemental folate intake[61]
61,433 women	14 years	↓ **40%** lower risk of intestinal cancer among women with the highest folate intake[62]
56,837 women	12 years	↓ **40%** lower risk of intestinal cancer among women with the highest folate intake[63]
61,433 women	15 years	↓ **34%** lower risk of intestinal cancer among women with the highest intake of vitamin B$_6$ ↓ **72%** lower risk of intestinal cancer among women who drink alcohol daily and have the highest intake of vitamin B$_6$[64, 65]
Meta-analysis of 7 studies	-	↓ **25%** lower risk of intestinal cancer with high folate intake, averaged across all studies[66]

Selenium lowers the risk of cancer

Why don't we get enough selenium?

Due to the flooding and leaching of soil during the Ice Age, the northern part of Europe, including Germany and France, constitute an area with selenium-deficient soils. On average, northern Europeans get 40–60 µg while 150–200 µg would be ideal. Just as with iodine, the low levels of selenium in the soil make it impossible to meet one's selenium needs naturally. In some countries fertilizers are enriched with selenium so that the deficiency can be combatted with selenium-rich grain.

Fighting cancer with selenium

Most of us don't know it, but we get cancer every day. Each day, damaged, degenerated cells are created in our bodies. Trace elements work in several ways to help destroy these cells – and not only preventively, but also once cancer cells have already developed.

It is thus no surprise to learn that the correction of our selenium deficiency has a significant effect on the occurrence of cancer. Selenium is an extremely important element in the prevention of cancer. This has been shown in more than 100 studies conducted on animals exposed to carcinogenic substances. 75% of these studies demonstrated a reduction in the frequency of cancer developing. (Remark: studies with carcinogenic substances can only be done with animals and even this, in my view, is unethical.)

GOOD TO KNOW

Selenium binds damaging substances
Selenium binds carcinogenic heavy metals, allowing them to be excreted from the body.

Optimum protection for cells
As part of the body's own antioxidant enzymes, selenium helps to intercept free radicals in the cells and thus prevents their mutation.

The immune system destroys cancer cells
Selenium stimulates lymphocyte activity (white blood cells) and killer cells. Studies show that intake of an additional 200 µg of selenium per day increases the activity of tumor-killing lymphocytes by 118%, and of killer cells by 82%.[67]

Selenium stimulates anti-cancer genes

Selenium blocks cancer cells

Selenium restricts cell division in cancer cells
↓

Selenium promotes apoptosis
Selenium can activate the "self-destructing" mechanism of cells

Selenium: Therapeutic use against prostate cancer

Responsible for nearly a quarter of all new diagnoses, prostate cancer is the most common cancer among men. You've certainly heard the word "chemotherapy" before. Today, the supplemental use of selenium is referred to as the first "chemo-preventive" strategy in the prevention of prostate cancer, and its usefulness is broadly accepted.

Micronutrients direct intelligent maintenance processes

Vitamin deficiency affects the likelihood of developing cancer. Over the course of millions of years of evolution, the best metabolic processes were selected: the ones which use the body's own repair processes to stop destructive changes in our cells and modifications to our genes, and which regulate them with a powerful and alert immune system. Micronutrients direct all these processes; that's what makes the optimal supply of these micronutrients so important.

Studies: Selenium against prostate cancer

Participants	Period	Results
9,345 men	20 years	↓ **51%** lower risk of prostate cancer among men with the highest levels of selenium in their blood[68]
58,279 men	6 years	↓ **31%** lower risk of prostate cancer among men with the highest levels of selenium in the toenails.[69] (Remark: trace elements are deposited in nails thus they may serve to analyse long term intake)
33,737 men	6 years	↓ **51%** lower risk of prostate cancer among men with the highest levels of selenium in the toenails[70]
Case control study of 1,163 men with prostate cancer compared with men without prostate cancer	-	↓ **48%** lower risk of prostate cancer among men with the highest levels of selenium in their blood[71]
5,141 men	8 years	↓ **41%** lower risk of prostate cancer among men taking supplemental selenium, vitamin C, vitamin E, and zinc[72]
Meta-analysis of 16 studies	-	↓ **26%** lower risk of prostate cancer with **any** supplemental intake of selenium, averaged across all studies. Higher selenium intake resulted in a greater risk reduction than the average.[73]

Dementia – the number 1 cause of the need for long-term care

What is dementia?

Dementia is the gradual loss of mental functions such as thought, memory, orientation, speech, and of learned abilities for everyday activities. The number of mentally handicapped older people is constantly on the rise. In Germany, about 1.2 million people are suffering from dementia, and that number is rapidly increasing. The reason: the risk of developing dementia increases with age. In the 65 to 69 age group, about one in 20 people have developed dementia, but in the 80 to 90 age group, it's nearly one in three. In 2010, it's predicted that 20% of all German citizens will be older than 65. Due to the rapid aging of society, experts predict 2.5 million dementia patients by the year 2030, and exploding costs of care of up to 40 billion euros annually. Currently, the US has about 4-5 million people with some form of dementia. In short, most countries in the developed world face a dramatic cost crisis of providing long-term care.

Both young and old are affected

What these numbers fail to reflect is what we can expect to face, both as a society and, especially, as individual families. Unlike other diseases, pharmaceutical costs are a very minor component of the cost of treating dementia. The true burden comes in the cost of care, and in the financial and emotional burdens on families, who carry out 85% of the care of dementia sufferers. As dementia progresses, the patient can hardly be left alone for even a moment. In the late stage, they need almost round-the-clock care: there's always the possibility that the patient might leave the stove alight and set the house on fire, or get lost in the city, or wander about on the street in a bathrobe, suffer sudden panic attacks or become aggressive, or stop practicing basic bodily hygiene. People suffering from dementia often feel themselves to be misunderstood, or get upset at being ordered around or patronized, as they're no longer capable of understanding why those taking care of them make the decisions they do. They often respond with anger when blamed for things they've long forgotten. Eventually, a complete loss of mental capacity may result.

Currently, there are too few daycare facilities for the care of patients in the early stages of dementia. Why would they be necessary? Because the families need a break. Many loved ones of dementia sufferers can hardly get out of the house, and end up devoting all of their time to caring for the patient, making it impossible for them to keep a job. This financial burden is exacerbated by the cost of paying for carers, daycare facilities, or nursing homes.

Is it possible to lower the risk of dementia?

Given these tragic family tales, it should be of great importance to everyone to know whether there is a way to protect the brain with antioxidants and vitamins, and perhaps reduce the likelihood of developing dementia. Interestingly, the first changes to brain tissue that typify dementia start to appear in young adults, and then increase with age. The actual onset of dementia occurs only once a significant proportion of brain cells have been destroyed.

How do vitamins work?

Vitamins protect nerves and blood vessels in the brain in several ways. Roughly speaking, there are two causes for the degeneration of the brain:

Nerve damage:
Causes may include Alzheimer's disease, nerve-damaging chemicals, or a shortage of nutrients for nerve growth.

Vascular system damage:
Affecting the vessels supplying the brain, caused by several small strokes or general damage to the brain's vascular system.

How B-vitamins protect the nerves
Building up nerve tissue:
Folate and vitamins B_6 and B_{12} are needed for the constant regeneration of neurons, or nerve cells. Dementia involves a loss of brain cells. Low levels of folate and vitamin B_{12} in the blood are an independent risk factor.

Production of quick-acting messenger subtances:
Folate, vitamins B_6 and B_{12} are used in the production of neurotransmitters such as acetylcholine, which are responsible for the rapid transmission of signals in the brain. In Alzheimer's patients, less and less of these messenger substances are produced over time, resulting in a decline in mental performance. In the studies, low folate levels in the blood go hand-in-hand with such declines in

mental functioning.

Protection against nerve damage:
Folate, vitamins B_6 and B_{12} break down homocysteine. The homocysteine molecule directly damages the nerve cells. Therefore, high homocysteine is a separate risk factor. People with high homocysteine levels run twice the risk of developing dementia or Alzheimer's.

Vitamin B deficiency and the consequences
90% of the population has a folate deficiency. The vitamin B_{12} deficiency is so great in the elderly over the age of 65 that even the conservative German nutritional society (DGE) recommends the use of vitamin B_{12}. Although the elderly have vitamin B_{12} in their diet, they have a poor uptable of this vitamin into the blood stream due to the aging colon. This results in an extreme B_{12} deficiency.

B-vitamins are active in building nerve tissue, in the production of neurotransmitters for greater cognitive performance, and they protect nerve cells against homocysteine.

Is it really still surprising that studies repeatedly show a direct correlation between low vitamin-B levels or high blood homocysteine levels and dementia? Over the course of evolution, our metabolism has developed a specific, necessary manner and degree of vitamin intake. This cannot be achieved with highly processed food products.

B-vitamins protect against damage to the vascular system
Protection against strokes.
Folate, vitamin B_6 and B_{12} break down homocysteine. High homocysteine increases the risk of stroke 4-fold. Several small, often unnoticed strokes are among the main causes for changes and losses in brain function. During a stroke the brain receives less oxygen and therefore large areas die off. Surely in your circle of acquaintances you have seen patients after a stroke and observed how slow these people become as a result of brain damage.

Protection against vascular damage.
Homocysteine directly damages the small blood vessels in the brain. This can lead to a decreased blood flow and to a lower supply of nutrients to certain areas of the brain. Especially folate, vitamin B_6 and B_{12} reduce the vascular-damaging homocysteine.

How do vitamin studies function with dementia?

First of all, it is remarkable that there are for fewer participants in the respective dementia studies. There are usually only between 100-800 participants, compared to 40,000 and more in cancer studies. Why is that? Cancer studies record the number of cancer cases for example breast cancer, and evaluates this statistically, along with vitamin blood levels or dietary records.

Study: The risk for dementia and Alzheimer's disease increases with low folate- or vitamin-B_{12} levels or with high homocysteine.

Participants	Period	Results
816 seniors, average age 74	4 years	↑ double the risk of developing dementia or Alzheimer's disease with high homocysteine levels ↑ double the risk of developing dementia or Alzheimer's disease with low folate bloodlevels[74]
370 Seniors, 75 and up	-	↑ double the risk of developing Alzheimer's disease with low folate- or vitamin-B_{12} bloodlevels[75]
650 men and women, average age 67	6 years	↑ the risk of the loss of cognitive performance increases parallel with increased homocysteine levels[76]
Overview analysis of over 24 studies with 4,486 participants	-	11 studies show that low folate blood levels and 9 studies show that low vitamin B_{12} blood levels are associated with less mental performance and dementia. Elaborate mental tests were carried out for this.[77]
965 men and women, 65 and up	6 years	↓ **50%** less risk of Alzheimer's disease in the group with the highest folate intake[78]

In contrast, in dementia studies very complex mental performance tests

THE NUN STUDY

In animals, one can determine all laboratory conditions in great detail. Food, temperature, way of life... There are few experimental setups where this can be done with people. But precisely this controlled type of experiment is particularly interesting for studies. In this book you will find some of these studies, like those of soldiers in Canada, vitamin C and colds (page 63), and also a study with prison inmates and vitamin B-withdrawal (page 71). For dementia, an interesting study was conducted with nuns in a convent, which shows the relationship between folate intake and dementia.[79] For decades, the sisters lived and worked together and ate from the same kitchen. Among the 30 nuns, who were between the ages of 78-101, the blood values were collected and after death a brain autopsy was performed. Please do not ask me how they were able to get nuns to agree to an autopsy. The result: the nuns had low folate blood levels, and also a significant reduction in brain cell mass of the neocortex ratio and increased Alzheimer's damage.

are conducted with each participant to determine a possible loss of brain functions: language tests, short-term memory tests, spatial reasoning, logical thinking and physical coordination. This is extremely expensive. One needs at least one hour per subject. Accordingly, these high-quality studies are carried out with a smaller number of participants.

Depression and vitamin deficiency

Depression is often the harbinger or typical symptom before dementia sets in. It is interesting that the production of nerve messengers (neurotransmitters) depends on B-vitamins. For example, the lack of serotonin triggers depression. The ability to learn and the short-and long-term memory also depends on these neurotransmitter substances, without them information cannot reach the brain. Depression or mood swings are therefore often a symptom of a bad B-vitamin supply. The risk of depression doubles with correspondingly low folate- and vitamin B_{12} blood levels (studies page 69). B-vitamin deficiency resulting in reduced nerve repair, high neurotoxic homocysteine levels and a 4-fold increased risk of stroke, is an important co-factor in the developement of dementia.

This is how vitamin C and E protect the nerve- and vascular systems

- Protection against free radicals: these can directly damage the nervous tissue. Vitamin C and E provide long-term protection for the 100 billion neurons in the brain.
- Free radicals and Alzheimer's: the most common cause of mental decline is Alzheimer's disease. One of the causes of the onset of Alzheimer's disease are free radicals.
- Protection against stroke: vitamins C and E reduce the risk of stroke and therefore, of course, the risk of brain damage.

Risk factor of vitamin deficiency

There are some studies that show no improvement in the prevention of dementia with the use of vitamins. However, these studies were usually conducted during far too short a period of time. This has nothing to do with long-term prevention. No single study, however, shows deterioration from the use of vitamins. There are so many positive studies on vitamins and the reduced risk of dementia, that you should not ignore this protection. Again, here the risk factor is the vitamin deficiency and not the intake of vitamins.

Study: Vitamin C and E decrease free radicals and strokes

Participants	Period	Results
5,395 men and women, average age 68	6 years	↓ **43%** less risk of the development of Alzheimer's disease with the participants with the highest vitamin E intake. ↓ **34%** less risk of the development of Alzheimer's disease with the participants with the highest vitamin C intake.[80]
4,740 men and women, 65 and up	5 years	↓ **64%** less risk of Alzheimer's disease with additional vitamin C and E intake.[81]
3385 men and women, age 71-93	8 years	↓ **70%** less risk of dementia in men who took vitamin C and E.[82]
894 men and women, 65 and up	5 years	↓ **50%** less risk of a loss of cognitive performance with additional intake of vitamin C and E.[83]

The osteoporosis-avalanche – second most common cause for long term care

Osteoporosis as a cause of death?

At first this would sound surprising. In fact, for women the risk of death from osteoporosis-related fractures is higher than the risk of dying from breast cancer. One in three women suffers at least one osteoporosis-related bone fracture. Every sixth woman suffers a severe fracture. About one-third of these patients died within the first 6 months thereafter. 20% needed long-term care. In comparison, "only" every ninth woman is diagnosed with breast cancer. Bad enough, but over the years the treatment of breast cancer treatment has made great progress.

Osteoporosis in numbers

The WHO (World Health Organisation) counts osteoporosis as one of the ten most important diseases around the globe. In the rapidly aging western societies the osteoporosis avalanche rolls with enormous costs. Already, the German health care costs of osteoporosis stands at 10 billion euros per year! The crazy thing is that osteoporosis is completely avoidable. In Germany, 6.5 million women and 1.3 million men are affected by osteoporosis. In the U.S. more than 40 million people either already have osteoporosis or are at a high risk due to low bone mass.

Loss of bone mass

During menopause a massive decline in minerals in the bones occurs because of the change of the hormonal system. Up to 40% of bone mass is lost with the resulting osteoporosis. First, you mostly lose body height. A "dowager's hump" and a curved spine are typical of this. Smaller vertebral fractures can lead to extremely painful back problems. 2.5 million Germans have already experienced such vertebrae fractures. Tooth loss is also often caused by osteoporosis. The small jaw bone where the teeth are anchored is the bone that will wear out the fastest and must therefore be constantly renewed. Rib fractures are also typical and can occur even when sneezing because of increasingly brittle bones. One "crumbles", say many patients. Then at some point the dangerous femoral neck and pelvic fractures occur; 130,000 per year in Germany. This then becomes the nursing care- or death sentence for many otherwise healthy patients that often are free of cardiovascular disease, diabetes or cancer.

The bone density measurement

Have your bone density measured every 3-4 years after menopause. One does not notice osteoporosis or the precursor osteopenia for many years, until it is too late. The health care system is absurd: the health insurance companies in Germany cover the bone density measurement tests only after the first osteoporotic fracture.

That's about as idiotic as measuring the blood fats after the first myocardial infarction. The measurement costs only 40 euros. Ideally, everyone should have this bone density test every 5 years after menopause.

Your bones - a large building site

Your bones are constantly assembled and disassembled. Like a huge road construction project, 5 million construction workers are constantly busy demolishing worn bone material, milling it away and recovering it with brand new bone. Why? Bones constantly experience fine micro cracks, which must be sealed and repaired just like busy highway bridges that receive regular repairs. The demolition squad (osteoclasts) eat old and torn mass away from bone. In this way, 400 mg of calcium and collagen bone fibres are milled away daily. By contrast, the construction crews are commanded by 20 different hormones and desperately need raw materials such as calcium, magnesium, zinc and vitamin D, C and K, which together ensure calcium absorption and its incorporation into the bone.

Age	Current calcium intake by women	This is how much calcium is recommended in Germany	This is how much additional calcium the average German needs daily
4-8 years	☹ 609 mg	800 mg	↑ 191 mg
9-13 years	☹ 707 mg	1300 mg	↑ 593 mg
13-19 years	☹ 785 mg	1300 mg	↑ 415 mg
19-50 years	☺ 780 mg	1000 mg	↑ 220 mg
50-65 years	☻ 890 mg	1200 mg	↑ 310 mg
65-80 years	☻ 813 mg	1200 mg	↑ 387 mg

Self-inflicted Osteoporosis – the calcium deficiency

Your bones need the building material calcium. A survey of 74,000 households[84] showed: 95% of Germans have a calcium deficiency.

Your bone structure needs vitamins

However, calcium alone has little success. Some studies actually show a decrease of bone fractures[85], but many large studies (over 115,000 men and women) show no change in the frequency of bone fractures.[86,87] Calcium does increase bone density, however, it does not increase the fracture resistance of the bones. You need a lot of organic materials to build unbreakable bones. Above all, vitamins K, C and D are needed for bone formation. The studies on these vitamins show a clear reduction in the risk of fractures.

Vitamin D for healthy bones

Vitamin D enhances calcium absorption in the intestines, decreases the excretion of calcium, fixes calcium in the bones and affects the endocrine system that controls the calcium incorporation in particular. Without vitamin D, calcium is almost worthless. 99% of Germans have too little vitamin D. While in the U.S. milk is often fortified with vitamin D, this is not the case in many countries. Vitamin D is formed by sunlight on the skin. Between October and March, the solar light spectrum in Germany is already too limited to stimulate vitamin D production in the skin. Germany is too far north on the globe for this, on the 45th degree of latitude. Again, it is logical: over the course of evolution humans and animals were outside all day and thus produced enough vitamin D for bone metabolism themselves. The office worker was not a foreseen evolutionary species.

TIP

Vitamin D and calcium are absolutely needed to build your bones. 90% of Germans have a vitamin D deficiency. During the winter months it is very important that adults take 400-800 IE of vitamin D and children take 500-1000 IE of vitamin D. Especially the elderly need vitamin D, as they do not have as much vitamin D build-up in their skin and often stay inside more.

Study: Additional vitamin D decreases the risk for osteoporosis

Overview analysis of 25 studies	Vitamin D against osteoporosis. With vitamin D, fewer bone fractures occur than with calcium alone: ↓ 37% less risk of vertebral fractures ↓ 23% less risk of femoral neck factures[88]
72,337 women	High vitamin-D intake over 18 years is compared to lower vitamin D intake: ↓ 37% less risk of vertebrae fractures[89]
Overview analysis of 29 clinical studies with 63,897 men and women	↓ 12% less risk for bone fractures of any kind with calcium and vitamin D intake ↓ 24% less risk in the group that has regularly taken high doses of calcium and vitamin D[90]
Overview analysis of 13 clinical studies with 19,114 men and women	Only high doses of vitamin D 700-800 IE, not low doses of 400 IE decrease the risk of fractures. ↓ 26% less risk of pelvic fractures[91]

Vitamin K for increased calcium incorporation

Vitamin K affects the bone building messengers and ensures that calcium is incorporated into the bones. Vitamin K is mostly found in green leafy vegetables and plants such as lettuce, broccoli, kale, etc. Today we no longer receive enough of these - at least not enough for our bone metabolism. Over the course of evolution over millions of years, vitamin K-rich plant foods were the basic diet. During the Stone Age we ate three times as many plant substances as we do today. In the U.S. in 2001 the recommended vitamin K intake was doubled[92] and is now twice as high as the recommendation of the German Nutrition Society (DGE). Actually there is no shortage of vitamin K, says the DGE. However, the DGE also knows that Germans rarely eat salad and fresh greens. Here again something does not fit together with the reference values - the way the argument runs is typical for nutrition societies worldwide.

Based on a three-times higher intake over the course of evolution, the analysis of the 7 studies with additional vitamin-K did not yield any surprises. They show that hip fractures can be reduced by 80%.

My tip: head for the salad bowls to protect your bones. Even old deer can still jump over trees without breaking their legs. Vitamin K makes this possible.

Caution: Bone terrorists

Smoking damages the bones. An overview analysis of 86 studies involving over 40,753 men and women shows: smoking increases the risk of hip fractures by 30-40%.[97]

Cortisone. Under cortisone treatment bone mass decreases rapidly. Bisphosphonates should be prescribed if you are on a longer cortisone therapy. These serve to rebuild the bone.

Drugs. There are various medications that strain your bones: thyroid hormones, anticoagulants, anti-epileptic drugs, diuretics, aluminium-containing gastric acid buffers.

Study: Eat more vitamin-K to protect against osteoporosis

72,327 women	↓ 30% less risk of femoral neck fractures with a higher vitamin-K intake.[93]
889 men and women	↓ 65% less risk of femoral neck fractures with a higher vitamin-K bloodlevels[94]
Overview analysis of 13 studies	↓ additional vitamin-K intake significantly decreases bone deterioration[95]
Overview analysis of 7 studies	With additional vitamin K ↓ 60% less risk of vertebral fractures ↓ 77% less risk of pelvic fractures ↓ 81% less risk of non-vertebral fractures[96]

Long-term protection of your eyes with antioxidants

With the example of your eyes I would like to show a further long-term insurance by way of antioxidants. You have been looking forward to your deserved retirement, and just when it is the time to read and travel, 20% of 65-year-olds and 40% of over 75-year-old suffer a terrible fate: macular degeneration.

This is how vitamin-C decreases the risk of macular degeneration[98]

Results: Decrease	Supplement	Participants	Study
↓ 45 %	Vitamin C	226	West (1994)
↓ 40 %	Vitamin C	390	Eye disease group (1993)
↓ 35 %	Vitamin C	876	Seddon (1994)
↓ 35 %	Vitamin C + E + Beta Carotene + Zink	2,587	AREDS Group (2001)

Protection of the macula with antioxidants

The macula, known as the yellow spot, is the sharpest point of vision in the eye. From here, 130 million photoreceptors guide visual information directly to the brain. A miracle of nature! This little spot concentrates the largest amount of stored antioxidants throughout the body, for the sole purpose of protecing the retina from damage caused by free radicals.

People with macular degeneration can unfortunately no longer read this text, because they suffer from a loss of central vision. Driving, reading, writing, watching TV - that and much more has become impossible. This leads to a shocking loss in quality of life. 2 million people in Germany suffer from the effects of macular degeneration. Vision loss is one of the most painful experiences in old age.

The damage to the macula can be successfully reduced by using antioxidants. Although vitamin C is only one of a total of approximately 10 stored antioxidants in the eye, vitamin C can reduce the occurrence of this disease in an impressive manner. Even with a dose of up to 2,000 mg vitamin C per day we can determine increases in the storage of this vitamin in the macula. Additional antioxidants and zinc can reduce the risk of macular degeneration by 35% (see table). In studies with over 118,000 participants, a diet with a high-fruit and -vegetable intake decreased the risk of macular degeneration by 64%.[99]

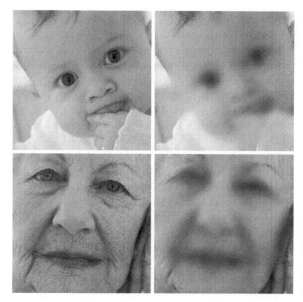

Loss of quality of life: Macular degeneration – not being able to see clearly in the central point of vision.

Protection against cataracts with antioxidants

In the U.S., each year 600,000 cataract operations are performed. 40,000 people are needlessly blind due to senile cataracts. To protect the eyes from damage caused by UV rays, the retina of the eye stores 30 times as much vitamin C as the adjacent tissue. The incidence of cataracts is decreased by 80% when high amounts of vitamin C and E and beta-carotene are found in the blood.[100] Important at this point: with beta-carotene intake we mean the intake of antioxidants from fruit and vegetables, not beta-carotene

GOOD TO KNOW

Protective substances for the eyes

Those who rely on the low German RDA-values of 90 mg vitamin C for males and 75 mg for females per day do not provide optimal protection for their eyes. The most important micronutrients fo the eye are the vitamins C, E, beta carotene, selenium and zinc. Above all, the phytochemicals lutein and zeaxanthin are deposited in the macula. Lutein is found in kale, spinach, brussels sprouts, broccoli, peas and pumpkin. Zeaxanthin is found in corn, tomato, carrots and many other vegetables.

pills. Compared to healthy people, cataract patients often have only 15% of the necessary selenium content in the blood and eyes.[101] Delaying cataract formation can prevent half of all cataract operations and significantly increase the quality of life of the elderly.[102]

Study: How antioxidants decrease the occurrence of cateracts[103]

Results: Decrease	Supplement	Participants	Study
↓ 50 %	Vitamin C 300-600 mg	350	Robertson et al. (1989)
↓ 40 %	Vitamin C	1,380	Leske et al. (1991)
↓ 45 %	Vitamin C 200 mg	50,800	Hankinson et al. (1992)
↓ 44 %	Multivitamins + Vitamin C	3,590	Sperduto et al. (1993)
↓ 40 %	Multivitamins + Vitamin C	2,151	Mares Perlmann (1994)
↓ 30 %	Multivitamins + Vitamin C	17,744	Seddon (1994)
↓ 30 %	Multivitamins + Vitamin C	4,300	Leske (1997)
↓ 41 %	Vitamin C	35,222	Yoshida (2007)
↓ 60 % 10 years	Vitamin C 360 mg	492	Taylor (2002)
↓ 77 % over 10 years	Vitamin C	247	Jaques et al. (1997)

Long-term protection and short time activation

What do you expect from vitamins? And how fast should they start working? In the long run, additional micronutrients and nutrition can reduce the risks of cardiovascular disease, cancer, osteoporosis, dementia and eye damage very effectively. It is THE very best insurance policy for your health.

Even in the short term you will already feel the benefits of the improved intake of vitamins with a more powerful immune system, a fitter metabolism. It makes you more efficient overall. Symptoms of an unexpected vitamin deficiency also often go away. The next chapter focuses on these issues.

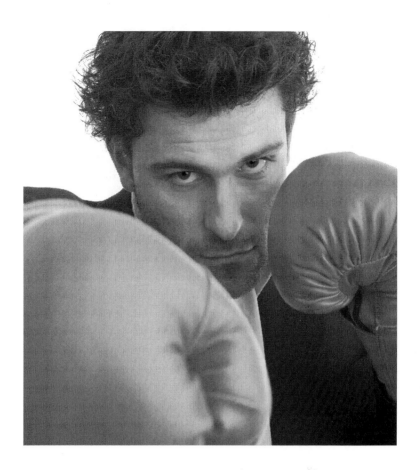

CHAPTER 3

Vitamins – for the immune system and a fitter metabolism

How do vitamins activate your immune cells? Why is vitamin C alone not enough for a well-functioning defence? Can vitamins reduce the frequency of a cold or shorten the duration of colds? The immune pharmacy – which vitamin intake is optimal during an infection? Why do vitamins improve your performance, your memory and your ability to learn? How do B-vitamins influence your psyche and mood?

A strong immune system

Daily guerrilla warfare

A whole army of bacteria and viruses, but also of abnormal cells (cancer) threaten your health every day. The immune system constantly wages a guerrilla war against these invaders. A war that is more immersive than any special coverage on CNN. Because all this does not happen thousands of miles away, but directly inside your own body. Did you know: you actually have cancer once a day. However, a powerful immune system removes the cancer cells and is the best protection against cancer.

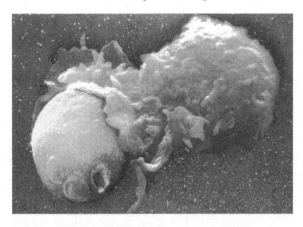

A powerful immune system: this cell of the immune system is armed with free radicals. These so-called macrophages ingest bacteria and foreign particles and dissolve them with free radicals.

Like a sniper in the war scenario, the killer cells and macrophages of the immune system fight bacteria and viruses first. When a macrophage ingests a bacterium, they bombard it with free radicals. With this attack it dissolves the cell walls of bacteria and can then destroy it. While the immune system is active, free radicals are produced and thus the need for antioxidants increases sharply. Do you have an idea what an immune cell looks like? The electron microscope shows an image in which a phagocyte swallows a bacterium to then dissolve it. You can immediately see the guerrilla war the immune system wages daily.

A fit immune system with vitamins

So that the produced free radicals do not destroy the macrophage itself, a lot of vitamin E is stored in its cell wall, which absorbs the free radicals there. Also for this reason, vitamin C is stored in the immune system in a 40-fold higher amount than in other cells.

In order to prevent self-destruction of immune cells in this immune system response, the immune system shuts down when insufficient amounts of vitamin C and vitamin E are available as free radical scavengers. This means that only when the immune cells are saturated with vitamin C does the defence work at full speed. Therefore, you should supply the immune cells with lots of antioxidants if you have an infection!

In order to defeat the multiplying virus millions of times, millions of immune cells have to be built at a very high speed. For this, muscle protein is quickly withdrawn from the body. B-vitamins are also needed for protein synthesis to build immune cells. In case of a B-vitamin deficiency the immune system is not very effective and powerful. With an infection one must hurry to provide the immune system with high doses of vitamins and rapidly available protein.

Vitamin C as a protection against colds

Humans are the only mammals that are unable to produce vitamin C in their intestines. A real "blunder" of evolution, which at the origin of this change (mutation) in the human genome did not have any negative effect, because the original food contained about 40 times more vitamin C compared to today's food! This was calculated by the two-time Nobel laureate Linus Pauling. In today's vitamin-poor diet it is a significant drawback for your immune system that it does not get enough vitamin C.

Immune cells saturated with vitamin C are more powerful in fighting viruses. It has been calculated that a cat produces between 10,000 and 15,000 mg of vitamin C daily. Humans, however, require external input of vitamin C for their immune system to become equally powerful. In spite of this the German Society for Nutrition (DGE) – which recommends a disproportionately low amount of 100 mg vitamin C daily – wonders why half of the German population catch colds in the winter time.

This amount of vitamin C helps to prevent infections in the winter time

Dozens of studies have confirmed clinical effects on the immune system. An example of an ideal control study was the administration of vitamin C to 112 Canadian soldiers living under identical conditions: same

> **GOOD TO KNOW**
>
> **Animals never catch colds.**
> The need for and consumption of vitamin C increases at times of infection. Animals increase this production in the intestine multiple times during these periods of time. This is the reason why animals never catch colds. The white blood cells become saturated with vitamin C and fend off viruses. The production of interferon, a transmitter which stimulates the defense mechanisms is also stimulated by vitamin C.[104]

sleeping quarters, same food, working under the same extreme conditions.[105] Administration of 1,000 mg of vitamin C daily reduced the frequency of catching colds by 68% compared to the control group who were not administered vitamin C.

As the phagocytic and killer cells function better with vitamin C, bacterial and viral infections can be fended off in advance. When everyone around you is ill in winter, the immune system can be optimized simply and inexpensively as a preventive measure.

This is how much vitamin C you need during an infection

In the case where a viral infection has already broken out, the amount of vitamin C intake must be increased substantially. An analysis of 20 vitamin C studies showed that 5,000 mg of vitamin C taken daily immediately when the infection starts, is the critical minimal dosage to shorten the period of infection by 25%. This is the dosage of vitamin C which you should take in the case of an acute infection.

For the immune system it makes a considerable difference if billions of viruses have to be destroyed after you have noticed the symptoms of a cold and then take high doses of vitamin C when it is much too late. If you take vitamin C at the beginning of the infection it can work powerfully against the relatively few viruses. This is effective before you even develop symptoms as the body can be prepared to prevent infection with sufficient vitamin C.

Protection from infection

Many underestimate to what extent the immune system can be reinforced through vitamins. It is very evident in the elderly who often have a weak immune system on account of a lack of micronutrients and are thus more prone to infection.[106, 107, 108] There is a study which provides impressive proof of this. The participants in the study were separated into two groups: group 1 were administered a multi-vitamin preparation and a fourfold dosage of vitamin E and beta carotene. Group 2 was administered a tablet containing no vitamins. The results were impressive.

- Over the course of a year the duration of the infection was 23 days in the group administered the vitamins and 48 days for the group which were not administered vitamins.
- The period in which antibiotics had to be administered was almost halved from 32 to 18 days!
- Blood tests showed greater killer cell activity and more phagocytes and T-cells which resulted in a direct improvement to the immune system.

This again shows clearly how vitamins stimulate the immune system and how important additional administration of them really is.

+++ SPECIAL: The first aid kit for infections +++

In the case of an infection, your immune system needs multiple amounts of micronutrients. Important: micronutrients work most effectively in a team. Multi-vitamin products and additional antioxidants lower the risk of infection better than vitamin C alone. Apart from this, the requirement of protein increase by 30% as millions of immune cells are produced which need protein as their construction materials. Even the need for glutamine even increases fivefold. This amino acid is used directly by the immune cells for cell division and as fuel. Taking aspirin in no way aids the immune system during infection. Aspirin increases the excretion of vitamin C tenfold. You need micronutrients and protein. This is the only means of keeping the immune system fit. When at home or when traveling you should always have micronutrients and protein available so you can act when you feel the first sign of symptoms. The following plan of action is recommended during an acute infection:

Micronutrients

- Take 5,000 mg of vitamin C immediately and top up again with 1,000 mg after a few hours. Vitamin C powder is acidic and can cause stomachaches. Vitamin C in a time-release formula is easier on the stomach.
- Take 400 mg of vitamin E daily. With vitamins E and C you are supporting the immune cells.
- Take a multi-vitamin tablet with B-vitamins three times daily. B-vitamins aid when immune cells are built from protein.
- Take 200 µg selenium once daily.
- Gargle with 20-60 mg zinc from effervescent tablets. The latter are particularly effective at the beginning of colds. Gargle as often as you can and put dissolved zinc on the nasal tissue using the little finger. Zinc hinders the viruses from docking on the mucous membrane. This reduces further infection of the mucous membranes and the immune system does the rest.

Protein and amino acids

- Take 80–100 g high-quality protein concentrate daily. 20 g of protein is equivalent to eating a whole steak. You can consume this amount by drinking several protein shakes daily.
- Take 25 grams glutamine. (2 heaped teaspoons) daily.

Vitamins save money

There is a popular public discussion in Germany that one of the many national holidays be done away with in order to stimulate the economy. But how about taking a serious approach to lowering the number of sick days annually? By this I do not mean that people should drag themselves to work in fear of being fired if they don't, but that the number of infections and sick days actually be reduced, thus saving labor costs. In this case vitamins really pay off. A study carried out in a medium-sized company on the frequency of colds and sick days for 54 employees over four winter months is an excellent example. Half of the employees received a high-dosed multi-vitamin and multi-mineral preparation. The other half were given a placebo – a tablet which has no effect.

In the group receiving vitamins the number of sick days was reduced from 8 to 2 days. In the group which did not receive vitamins the average number of sick days remained 8 days as in the previous year.[110] In the group which received vitamins one could identify an increase in the number and activity of immune cells. The company made a savings of 36,000 euros in four months due to the reduction of sick days.

Very similar results were obtained in a placebo-controlled study among 130 participants in the US. Again one group was given a multi-vitamin / multi-mineral preparation and the other a placebo. Here again sick days were reduced by more than half.[111]

Colds and influenza cost health insurance schemes one billion euro annually. The German economy would save several billion euro if workers had fewer sick days. But this requires investing some money in additional vitamins as well as a qualitative improvement in the catastrophic food offered in company cafeterias largely consisting of fatty, overcooked meals which are low in micronutrients. This does not strengthen the metabolism or provide the immune system with sufficient micronutrients.

Survive thanks to a potent immune system

40 million people died of the Spanish flu in 1918; that is more than the numbers killed in the 1st World War. Major fatal flu epidemics break out about once every ten years. Currently new scenarios are being calculated for new viruses such as the bird flu, which would spread rapidly due to today's mobility and air travel. It could quickly account for 100 million deaths. But the really significant detail is forgotten in the reports and newspaper articles. It is true that 40 million people died from the Spanish Flu but 500 million were affected. So only 10% of those with the infection died. Why did so many survive? It was the immune system of each individual which accounted for the difference. The stronger it is, the better the chances are of surviving the next

epidemic.

Vitamins strengthen your immune cells. In order to give you a rapid overview of the effects of vitamins on the immune system, you will find 91 studies on immune system and vitamins in the table below.[112] What is the use of such a table? The answer is simple: again and again acquaintances or the tabloid press unsettle you by insisting that additional vitamins have no effect. But in certain "regiments" of the immune system the effects of vitamins can be measured and proven. The defense system against infections and tumors only works with an immune system getting everything it needs. It is the cornerstone of your health.

How vitamins activate the cells of the immune system

Vitamins	T4-cells	Phago-cytes	Killer cells	Antibody response	Lympho-cyte repro-duction	B-cell activity
A	↑	↑	↑	↑	↑	
Beta carotin	↑	↑	↑		↑	
B_{12}	↑					↑
C		↑	↑			
E	↑	↑	↑	↑	↑	↑
Lack of vitamins causes						
B_6	↓	↓	↓	↓	↓	↓
A	↓	↓	↓		↓	

An optimized metabolism

How do you feel at the moment? How fast does your brain work? How strong is your stress resistance and how high will your performance level be in the coming hours? All this depends upon whether your body has the necessary micronutrients for your metabolism to run smoothly. B-vitamins are also called psychogenic vitamins as they exert a direct influence on your intellectual performance, your learning ability, your memory, your emotional state and your nervous resilience. Restlessness, aggression, sleep disturbances, inability to concentrate and a low stress tolerance level often is related to a lack of B-vitamins.

Mental stability and intellectual performance

There are a host of good examples of how B-vitamins affect the nervous system. For example, Vitamin B_1 plays a role in the transfer of nerve impulses in the brain. In addition, it helps to create the neurotransmitter acetylcholine ensuring that it is not broken down too quickly. It is only through acetylcholine that information can be stored in the memory. A lack of both substances reduces both memory retention and learning ability as the moist and oily film on the brain neurons becomes too dry.

Another example is vitamin B_3. In the case of a lack of vitamins a very rare protein building block – tryptophan - is transformed into vitamin B_3. Tryptophan is an indispensable component of the "happy hormone" serotonin. Through the lack of vitamin B_3 - a bottleneck for the production of serotonin is created. If rodents are deprived of B_3 and tryptophan, they quickly become extremely aggressive on account of the lack of serotonin. Even the smallest lack of this vitamin has immediate effects on the brain.

The biochemistry of feelings

Primarily it is the B-vitamins which are needed in the production of the nerve messengers – neurotransmitters. Serotonin, dopamine and norepinephrine are such neurotransmitters. Vitamin B_6 helps to create all structures containing protein, which are part of neurotransmitters. It is remarkable what power biochemistry has in influencing human emotions...

Norepinephrine is the neurotransmitter of champions

It makes us stress-resistant, self-confident and more concentrated. It motivates us to tackle problems with enthusiasm. The U.S. army has long used B-vitamins and certain amino acids (the components for protein) to ensure that soldiers under stress on monitoring equipment remain concentrated for longer periods of time. Many top managers also use protein and B-vitamins to increase their concentration levels.

Dopamine for a rush of happiness.

All drugs, whether ecstasy, cocaine, nicotine or alcohol affect the dopamine system. They prolong the presence of dopamine on the receptors of the nerves in the brain. Dopamine creates a sensation of euphoria, enthusiasm and a good mood. Fantastic that you can have this without drugs: for these real "happy messengers" you need protein and vitamins.

Serotonin for a balanced temperament

Serotonin is a relaxing "mood enhancer" in our brain and nervous system. Increased memory, good sleep, balanced mood; all this depends on serotonin. What does it feel like when you are stressed? You are in a filthy mood, do not sleep well and in mega-stress situations your memory lets you down. You forget the simplest things. In stressful situations increased quantities of B-vitamins and protein components are used for neurotransmitter production.

Depression and lack of vitamins

Low serotonin production due to of a lack of B-vitamins can bring your spirits and feelings to their limits. Depression in humans does not necessarily stem from external circumstances but is often biochemical in nature. In depressed people too low B-vitamin and tryptophane levels- the nutrient responsible for creating serotonin are often noted. Excessively high homocysteine values due to a lack of B-vitamin intake can also be ascertained. The lack of vitamin B is the bottleneck for the production of serotonin.

Antidepressants such as Prozac prolong the presence of serotonin in the brain. Of course this can be approached from the other side by ensuring a better production of serotonin. That is what nature has been taking care of for millions of years. Depressive moods can be influenced by vitamins B_1, B_3, B_6, B_{12}, folic acid [115, 116] and certain protein components (amino acids).

Studies: Depression and low folate or high homocysteine levels

Study participants	Result
924 males	↑ Doubles the risk of depression in males with the highest homocysteine values[113]
Overview analysis of 11 studies with 15,315 men and women	↑ 55% higher risk of depression with low folate values[114]

Premenstrual syndrome and B-vitamins

More women than men suffer from migraines and depression. Often this has more to do with the metabolism than one would think. 75% do not get the minimum quantity of the nerve vitamin B_6. Often the reasons for this are frequent diets, hormonal changes during their period and, not to be forgotten, taking the pill. The latter can reduce the level of vitamin B_6 in the blood by 20%. The resulting lack of B-vitamins causes extreme fluctuations in the production of serotonin. A third of all women between 30-40 years of age suffer from PMS, resulting in frequent depression, mood fluctuations and cravings for sweets – chocolate in particular. The body knows what is missing for chocolate contains some serotonin.

One of the causes of PMS is a combined lack of vitamins B_6, B_3 and tryptophane. When the hormone system changes - one week prior to a woman's period - more vitamin B_6 and B_3 are used up. For example, vitamin B6 is required actively on certain hormone receptors. At the same time more vitamin B_3 is produced from tryptophane, the irreplaceable constituent of the "mood enhancer" serotonin. In the meantime 9 studies have been made involving over 1,000 female participants[117], which show that PMS symptoms are reduced by between 40 and 80% through the daily administration of 50-200 mg of vitamin B_6. Tryptophane has also been shown to be an effective means of fighting PMS.[118] Additional B-vitamins and a protein shake daily containing tryptophane raise the serotonin level and work true miracles.

Hyperactive children - nutrients for the nervous system

An increasing number of parents are being confronted with the problem of hyperactive children. ADHD (Attention Deficit Hyperactivity Disorder) is big business for the pharmaceutical industry. Often it is treated much too soon with medication. The long term effects of this are not even known. Instead doctors should consider nutrient deficiencies first. In both Great Britain and the U.S.A. a therapeutic alternative with nutrients has been applied for many years. This can reduce the main symptoms by up to 20%. Even in severe cases medication can often be lowered. The "junk food generation" stuffs itself with calories but gets little nutrients for the nerves and the brain. Nutrients can often put the metabolism of hyperactive children on the right track again: more B-vitamins and magnesium for the nervous system, more protein for the neurotransmitters and, above all, as many omega-3 fatty acids as possible for the brain. Particularly in the crucial years of childhood, where the

THE REALITY SHOW WITH VITAMIN B WITHDRAWAL

Vitamins are a necessity of life. After just 4 weeks, withdrawal effects from a lack of B-vitamins become very apparent in the results of an experiment conducted by the University of Iowa on prisoners who were given a diet lacking vitamin B_6.

First week:

The prisoners suffered headaches and became either more aggressive or depressed; they were easily irritated or apathetic, unmotivated and tired. They had problems concentrating and had sleep disturbances. This after only one week? You have already noticed why: the neurotransmitters production is quickly affected. Symptoms of a slight lack of vitamin B_6 set in. Many of your fellow citizens with grim facial features may have this deficiency as well. It is a fact that three-quarters of citizens in affluent societies do not get sufficient quantities of vitamin B_6 in their diet.

Second week:

There was evidence of irritated, flaky skin, eczema, chapped lips. The reason: there already was an insufficient amount of vitamin B_6 for the production of protein for skin cells. These cells are renewed very frequently.

Third week:

The inmates got diarrhoea, nausea and vomiting. In addition, the protein storage area, i.e. the muscles - were depleted.

Fourth week:

Dramatic. Anaemia developed. The immune systems of the inmates collapsed with a rapid decrease in white blood cells, antibodies and killer cells. The experiment had to be cut short at this point.

The inmates were rewarded as promised with reduced periods of detention. This four-week "high-speed" test showed the effects of a lack of vitamin B_6. Without knowing it many people suffer to some degree from symptoms related to an insufficient intake of vitamin B_6. A moderate deficiency is quite often found in pregnant women and in the elderly. A severe lack of vitamin B_6 with the effects described is also found in the chronically and severely ill. But this experiment does show one thing, above all: the biochemically controlled metabolism suffers immediately from a deterioration in the supply of micronutrients.

academic performance of children decides their future, additional nerve and brain nutrients along with a well balanced diet are of paramount importance. This strategy can save parents a lot of stress.

In top form at the office

If you eat fatty junk food which is low in nutrients in the cafeteria and do not take additional vitamins, minerals and trace elements, you need not be surprised that both physically and mentally you are working at a slower pace. During the afternoon, almost paralyzed by the digestion of all the fatty food, you are often virtually only capable

> **TIP**
>
> You feel as well as your metabolism allows you to. If important micronutrients are lacking, the metabolism slows down. You become irritable, feel low and your performance drops. With micronutrients you can exert a major influence on your entire nervous system and your productivity.

of doing next to nothing. The protein from the fat-roasted pork takes at least 3-4 hours to reach the bloodstream. But whoever eats a light lunch and tops up with quickly absorbed protein from a protein shake and with vitamins can stimulate the neurotransmitters for intellectual performance and concentration. The alert brain, a stable nervous system and a good mood even when under stress is your competitive advantage over your colleagues whose metabolism is through the floor. You cannot even begin to imagine how often a metabolic problem is at the root of the stressed behavior of managers...

Would you fill up your Ferrari with heating oil?

One thing should be clear to everybody: if you fill up your Ferrari sports car with heating oil you will never reach top speed. Your human metabolic engine can only reach peak performance with the correct metabolic accelerators – micronutrients. As you already know the metabolic engine works like a conveyor belt in a factory in many individual assembly and processing steps which have to be completed in sequence. If a vitamin, a mineral or a trace element is missing at the outset, the conveyor belt (metabolism) will continually slow down.

+++ SPECIAL: Interview +++

Klaus Pietrzik is a professor at the Institute of Nutritional Science, at the University of Bonn. He is an internationally recognized expert in the field of B-vitamins and preventive medicine. With about 300 scientific publications he is one of the truly outstanding nutritional scientists.

Andreas Jopp: *What is the focus of your research? What makes vitamins so exciting?*
Prof. Pietrzik: I've been working at the Institute of Nutritional Science at the University of Bonn for 30 years now. The focus of my research are micronutrients - especially the B-vitamins. The exciting thing about vitamins is that even though they were discovered early last century, we are constantly discovering new effects. Previously vitamins were taken to prevent deficiency symptoms. Today prevention is more the focus. That is, to exploit the preventive effects that are associated with cardiovascular disease, but also with Alzheimer's disease and dementia.

Is the importance of the results from nutritional research related to obesity, blood pressure or cardiovascular disease adequately reflected in medical practice?
It usually takes 10 years to implement scientific findings into practice. Be aware that research first needs to become textbook knowledge. Take the example of homocysteine. I researched this field for 15 years, and only the newer textbooks of internal medicine address homocysteine, and then only a mere half of a page.

And what about the nutrition training of physicians?
Regrettably, the medical studies in Germany place too little emphasis on the basics of nutrition. Of course, the functions of vitamins are treated as part of basic studies. But in further medical training these important micronutrients are no longer addressed. Most practitioners do not quite know how individual vitamins work and what they are good for. Most doctors are not familiar with the newer nutrient studies. They mostly have a very general knowledge, for example that you should get enough vitamins in your diet. The patient should keep this in mind when he speaks with his doctor about vitamins and notices a negative attitude.

To what extent are we undersupplied with folate?
The entire population does not get enough folate. About half the population gets 75% less than the desired intake. This is simply because we do not eat 5

portions of fruits and vegetables a day; practically no one does.

Folate is mostly found in fruits and vegetables. In 1940 it was isolated in spinach leaves. "Folium" - Latin for "the leaf" - has given the vitamin its name.

90% of the population does not have the minimum folate intake. Is the claim of the German Society for Nutrition (DGE) to re-educate the population, not very unrealistic?
That is absolutely correct. Because folates in food are very sensitive. Folates are destroyed during cooking and storing. This is different with synthetic folic acid, which is absolutely stable. So when food is fortified with it, folic acid is not destroyed during food preparation or baking.

However, nature did not intend for us to be nutrient-deficient and nature did not intend that we have to go to pharmacies. On the other hand, there are foods that are folate-rich but that we do not eat for other reasons. For example, liver is the most folate-rich food, but due to pollution and high vitamin A content, the regular consumption of liver was discouraged.

Even the DGE itself admits that it is "almost impossible for women to receive the required amount of folate with a normal diet"[119] Even in children you cannot manage this without enrichment. Should women between 14-45 take additional folic acid?
With such a deficiency, one cannot help but think seriously about folic acid enrichment. This is now required in more than 30 countries. In the U.S., Canada, Brazil and Chile, it has already been implemented into laws. Europe, Austria, England and Ireland are facing the introduction of enrichment in staple foods. In Germany it is only being discussed, but it has not been implemented into practice.

How many children are aborted due to a neural defect or will be born with it due to folate deficiency?
700-1400 neural tube defects are projected per year in Germany. About half of them are detected early, and then, after appropriate education and subsequent explanation and agreement a possible abortion is initiated. Many cases are not detected. And from that you can extrapolate that about 400-500 children are born with severe disabilities and require lifelong care.

Counted over 10 years, Germany could have had 14,000 more children and 14,000 fewer family tragedies with a few micrograms of folic acid. The enrichment of staple foods and education are urgently needed!

Leaflets of dietary supplements are not allowed to contain research results from

studies or make claims about the effects of vitamins, even though worldwide, important vitamin studies were conducted that would justify statements.
It would certainly make sense to provide more information about vitamins in the leaflets. On the other hand medical statements would require vitamins to become approved drugs. Again, for this costly, studies are needed, money that no pharmaceutical company would spend on an unpatentable vitamin.

An adequate vitamin – or folate – intake decreases the risk of cardiovascular disease in the healthy...
Yes, this was shown by several studies from the U.S.A. and Canada. Here staple foods have been enriched with folic acid since 1998. The results also show that within a few years there was a statistically significant decrease in the number of strokes. This data is based on a population of at least 250 million people.

In the prevention of cardiovascular disease in healthy people, extra folic acid is effective. I've always felt that patients who already have a disease overestimate the potential of vitamins to repair damage. Vitamins are more effective in the prevention of diseases rather than as therapeutic drugs.
I can confirm that. But there are interesting studies, for example, those that deal with deposits in the arteries. It was shown that vitamin intake can lead to a reduction in deposits. Other studies show that the vessel wall thickness is better with a folic acid supplementation than with a placebo. It is entirely conceivable that vitamins still generate positive effects even with patients who are already ill.

There is much debate about whether we need a lot of B–vitamins. Genetic factors, diseases, medications and many others things can greatly increase the vitamin requirements. The homocysteine level is very interesting. If it is too high, then one should no longer discuss the pros and cons of vitamins. The cause behind it is most often a deficient intake of the relevant B–Vitamins. Conclusion: thoroughly revise eating habits and possibly take vitamins.
Yes, homocysteine levels can be measured as an indicator of an adequate vitamin-B intake and as a risk factor for various diseases. Homocysteine levels can be reduced very effevtively with folate and vitamin B_{12}.

What is the proper homocysteine level?
The homocysteine level in healthy individuals without risk factors is tolerable up to 12 micromol. For people over 60 years of age or those with risk factors, the value should not exceed 10 micromol.
Do doctors take the homocysteine levels into consideration?

More doctors know the importance of homocysteine levels now then 10 years ago, but few use it therapeutically and reduce it with B-vitamins.

That is similar with the lipid-lowering effect of vitamin B_3. Pharmaceutical companies have always preached to physicians that vitamin B_3 does not work. Therefore, it was rarely used. Meanwhile, the first lipid lowering agents were combined with vitamin B_3 in a tablet.
Yes, exactly.

Another focus of your work is the relationship between B-vitamins and cognitive decline - dementia - in old age. Are the elderly generally B_{12} deficient and can vitamins be preventive here?
Both. The problem is the following: up to 30% of over 60-year-olds develop gastritis. The pH in the stomach increases. Then it is no longer possible to disolve and absorb vitamin B_{12} from the protein binding. This way, many develop a vitamin B_{12} deficiency, even if they receive B_{12} with their normal food intake. It therefore really makes sense to give the eldery vitamin B_{12} supplements. The experts agree on this.
The United States is now considering also enriching foods with vitamin B_{12} in addition to folic acid. That makes sense, because folic acid and B_{12} are involved together in the homocysteine metabolism, and the elderly often lack both. This leads to elevated homocysteine levels, and these are responsible for the progression of vascular damage, also in the brain.

And how does this work exactly?
As a result, there is damage to the small vessels in the brain. This leads to a decreased blood flow, which also means a reduced supply of nutrients. This leads to microinfarcts with a corresponding loss of mental capacity. This limitation in intellectual capacity that originates in the vascular system is difficult to distinguish from the constraints of Alzheimer's disease. Apparently, both processes run parallel.

Aside from dementia, depression also plays a major role in the elderly. B-vitamin deficiency and neurotransmitters are closely related....
The B-vitamins are involved directly in the production of neurotransmitters. In addition, B-vitamins are necessary for the production of choline, acetylcholine, thus for the building blocks of nerve tissue and nerve conductors. Accordingly, it is not surprising that in a deficiency, corresponding failures can be observed.

What impact do B-vitamins have on performance?

We are currently investigating, whether additional B-vitamins lead to better physical performance in athletes. We have published the first positive results, which show that performance optimization can be achieved with that.

How is it that in the press one more often reads negative than positive news headlines about vitamins?
As a neutral scientist I am quite asthonished about the media. In particular the speed with which news is spread when there is a negative result in a vitamin study. For example, the NORVIT study: a press conference was called immediately and it was said that the homocysteine theory was dead. Not two days later did the newspapers report on it. On the same day, however, there also appeared a report from North America, which showed that there was a significant reduction in strokes due to folic acid enrichment of certain foods. This was not reported to the public. It is surprising that negative results are published first, and always get corresponding press coverage. Hardly anyone is interested in positive results, and the general reader may not know or recognize this, of course.

Yes, one can indeed observe a general tendency that the risk of overdose of B-vitamins is always stressed more than for example the positive effect on cardiovascular disease.
Which is utter nonsense of course. Overdoses of vitamin B_{12} are unknown. Furthermore, an overdose of folic acid is completely non-toxic. The only thing that was described in the scientific literature for 50 years was that when taking high doses of folic acid the symptoms of a B_{12} deficiency can be masked. This was last observed in the 1950's, when folic acid was still taken in extremely high doses. Nobody takes such doses. Since then, the scientific literature have published no more reports about this. So it is very doubtful to peddle such arguments and to say that B-vitamins are dangerous.

Also, an excess of B-vitamins would be excreted in the urine without any problems...
Yes. With vitamin B_6 one can still argue about where the line is. But for the healthy it really doesn't make sense to take more than two to three times the recommended daily allowance of vitamin B_6. If one takes it 20-fold, well okay, then you may consider whether there are unwanted side effects.

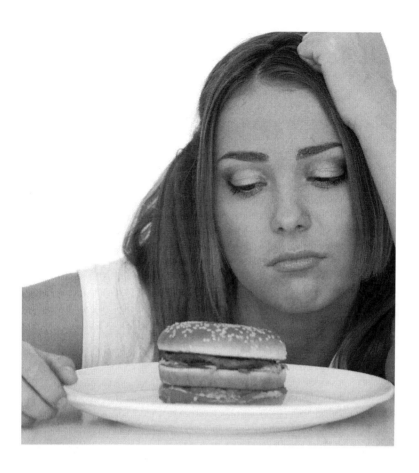

CHAPTER 4

Deficiency in affluent societies

Do large parts of the population really have a vitamin deficiency? What do typical symptoms of vitamin deficiency feel like? What amount of vitamins is lost during the processing and storage of food? Why do we have fewer vitamins now than during the time of early evolution? Why are vitamin intake recommendations often outdated and do not correspond with an optimal intake for disease prevention? What can you expect from vitamins? When are the effects of vitamins overrated?

Micronutrient deficiency - the majority

What do you think: do you get the minimum requirement of vitamins?
Like the majority of people, you will answer this question with a "yes".

What is the reality? Studies with more than 80,000 participants from Germany, France and the United States, where the shopping and eating behavior was studied, show that 80% of the population does not even get the minimum requirement of vitamins which are needed to prevent deficiency symptoms.

Perhaps you are one of the 20%, who by eating an exceptionally healthy diet, meets these minimum requirements. But even then with our current foods, you will under no circumstances achieve the optimal intake of vitamins which is necessary for the prevention of cancer and cardiovascular diseases. The intake for a functioning metabollism which we had during the time of the evolution is not archieved nowadays.

What does "recommended daily allowance" (RDA) actually mean? What do the big studies on nutritional behavior and the health outcomes actually show? What can you learn from these?
As an example, the German Society for Nutrition (DGE) gives extremely low daily intake recommendations (reference values) for vitamins and minerals for the prevention of deficiency symptoms. These amounts should be achieved by all segments of the population through their diet. This minimum requirement is the lower limit - let's say the vitamin basis that any prisoner should receive. It does not include an increased need due to special circumstances such as age, growing phase, pregnancy, disease, smoking, alcohol or drugs use.

High micronutrient-deficiency in the population

Five major nutrition studies from three highly developed countries show that, despite the low minimum intake values, the majority of the population is not sufficiently supplied with vitamins, minerals and trace elements. How good is the vitamin-intake really?

INFO

The minimal allowance values do not represent the best possible care. Many experts agree on this. An optimal supply may be around 3x the RDA as it was during the time of evolution.

The Germans - an abundance of deficiency

In the National Nutrition Survey in Germany (Vera) 23,000 chosen consumers participated. In women between the ages of 19 and 35 a deficiency was detected:

- In 49% for vitamin C
- In 66% for vitamin B_{12}
- In 99% for folate
- In 90% for vitamin D
- In 76% for vitamin B_6

Regarding folate, zinc, iodine and calcium hardly any German receives the already low minimum values which are recommended by the German Society for Nutrition. For selenium no guideline is even set. With the German diet the selenium-deficiency cannot be covered anyway due to depleted soils. The metabolism and the immune system of many Germans starve at full tables.

The American fast-food society

In the U.S.A., 21,500 participants took part in a study by the Ministry of Agriculture.[120] None, I repeat, **none** of the 21,500 participants achieved the minimum intake recommended by RDA values for the vitamins A, B_1, B_2, B_6 and B_{12} as well as calcium and iron. People who eat junk food or highly processed foods even only once a day have little chance to achieve the minimum RDAs. While one would think that obese Americans are well nourished, they are actually completely undernourished with vital nutrients at a cellular level.

France- this is how good the French actually eat

In France, three large representative studies were conducted: ESVITAF, the Food Consumption Study in Burgundy and the Study in Val de Marne. These three studies show that even our gourmet loving neighbors do not receive the recommended minimum values through their diet. Dr. Curtay showed what percentage of the population does not achieve the vitamin and mineral recommendations and summarized the three studies in the table next page.[121] The RDAs represent the minimum requirements for micronutrients. The large consumption studies show that these days even this lower value is barely

> **GOOD TO KNOW**
>
> **Minimal intake is barely achieved**
> The RDAs are your minimum requirements for micronutrients. The large consumption studies show: even this lower requirement is barely achieved. It is no wonder then that this deficiency leads to the various symptoms of micronutrient deficiency that are suffered by so many without being aware of the cause.

reached. The French, like all northern Europeans, eat food where 35-40% of the calories come from fat. However, fat contains almost no micronutrients. So even in a French paradise you cannot achieve the minimum supply.

Percentage of the population that does NOT receive the recommended minimum vitamin values through their diet (based on the results from the three studies in France[122, 123, 124])

Vitamin-/Mineral deficiency	Men	Women
↓ A	12-60%	9-50%
↓ B₁	43-80%	69-80%
↓ B₂	27-60%	24.6-60%
↓ B₃	49.5%	49.3%
↓ B₆	67.5-80%	90-92%
↓ Folate	40-90%	50-90%
↓ C	25-60%	15-60%
↓ D	90-98%	90-98.6%
↓ E	40-100%	75-100%
↓ Calcium	20%	30%
↓ Iron	5%	55-90%
↓ Magnesium	60%	80%
↓ Zinc	80%	90%
Selenium	90%	90%

Why experts are taking micronutrients

For optimal intake, many experts recommend at least 3 times the values recommended by the RDA. If the RDAs were to be revised (upwardly), an even greater proportion of the population would have a distinct deficiency. But then this would also mean that the recommendation for a "diverse Western" diet would no longer be sufficient.

INFO

RDA-US and RDA-EU are the U.S. and the European minimum intake levels for micronutrients. You often find the term RDA on the label of multivitamins. For example, a vitamin tablet contains B₃, and the respective percentage of the RDA minimum requirement.

Most experts have long been aware of this fact: a survey by the magazine Prevention with the most respected nutrition scientists showed that they take vitamin supplements almost without exception. Nutrition experts especially take vitamin C at a dose of 500-3000 mg daily. This value is 6 to 40-fold above the RDA.[125]

Dr. Burton Kallman of the National Nutritional Food Association has calculated that for the standard diet of monkeys in U.S. zoos the recommended values are 23 times higher than what the RDA recommends for people.[126] Our closest relatives need that many vitamins in order to maintain their health, to protect themselves against infection and to procreate at the zoo. The genetic material of monkeys differs just 1% from our genetic material.

Vitamin deficiency and deficiency symptoms

Look at the table on the next page, which shows the typical symptoms of vitamin deficiency and the proportion of the population that does not meet the minimum values for these vitamins. You will immediately notice: both have something in common. Even as a doctor you might get this: if 90% of the population has a deficiency for vitamin D and folate, this will most likely have consequences and symptoms.

In vitamin deficiency there is always a whole range of symptoms, which at first glance do not seem related. Doctors, however, are more trained to locate symptoms of certain diseases. It is unusual for them to suspect a vitamin C deficiency when observing a combination such as bleeding gums, susceptibility to infection and fatigue. Or to blame dry skin and night blindness plus retinal problems on a vitamin A deficiency. Or relate a B-vitamin deficiency to depression. Instead, too often medications are prescribed without knowing the true cause of the problem, which too often are improper nutrition and micronutrient deficiencies.

INFO

We get sick due to our diet and want to be made healthy by medicine. Medicine has become an expensive repair shop due to suboptimal nutrition.

Do you suffer from a vitamin deficiency? If you have several typical symptoms, then you may have a vitamin deficiency.

Micro-nutrient	What are these micronutrients needed for?	Typical deficiency symptoms and long-term consequences	Percentage of the population in the three French studies who did not achieve the minimum intake
Vitamin B₁	Nerve-, muscle and carbohydrate metabolism, neurotransmitter synthesis	↑ Irritability, ↑ Difficulty concentrating, ↑ Insomnia, ↑ Depression, ↑ Irregular heart rhythm, ↑ Fatigue, ↑ Headaches, ↑ Susceptibility to infection	↓ 43-80%
Vitamin B₆	Protein metabolism, growth processes, immune system, neurotransmitters	↑ Depression, ↑ Restlessness, ↑ Premenstrual syndrome, ↑ Irritability, ↑ Scaly skin, ↑ Frequent infections	↓ 67-90%
Folate / Folic acid	Bloodformation, Immune system, neurotransmitters	↑ Fatigue syndrome, ↑ Depression, ↑ Irritability, ↑ Forgetfulness, ↑ Insomnia, ↑ Long-term decreased immunity, ↑ Cardiovascular disease, ↑ Dementia, ↑ Cancer, ↑ Osteoporosis	↓ 50-90%
Vitamin C	Involved in 15,000 metabolic reactions, immune system, formation of connective tissue, fat burning, construction of important hormones and neurotransmitters, antioxidant	↑ Susceptibility to allergies, ↑ Bleeding gums, ↑ Susceptibility to infection, ↑ Fatigue, ↑ Long-term poor fat burning, ↑ Cardiovascular diseases, ↑ Risk for cancer, ↑ Cataracts (grey star), ↑ Blood pressure	↓ 25-60%

Micro-nutrient	What are these micronutrients needed for?	Typical deficiency symptoms and long-term consequences	Percentage of the population in the three French studies who did not achieve the minimum intake
Vitamin E	Antioxidant, protects cell membranes and the retina; prevents oxidation of blood fats	Long-term: ↑ Cancer ↑ Cardiovascular disease ↑ Cataracts	↓ 40-100%
Vitamin A / Beta-Carotene	Function of the cell membranes, eyes, skin and mucous membranes	↑ Night blindness ↑ Cancer ↑ Dry skin ↑ Nervousness ↑ Retinal problems	↓ 12-60%
Vitamin D	Bone structure, calcium absorption, immune system, cell proliferation	↑ Fatigue ↑ Irritability ↑ Long term susceptibility for infection ↑ Osteoporosis ↑ Cancer	↓ 90-98%

Treatment of the symptoms – we all pay for the costs

For a vet, an analysis of the food always comes first. Only after that are drugs used. That should also be done with humans: a weight and diet survey, a blood test for different micronutrients and oxidative stress. People who are overweight have fuelled their cells badly with mostly fat, sugar and highly refined foods. First, one needs to compensate the deficiencies, which will slowly balance your metabolism before returning to the symptoms. That should be the rule.

A symptom is like a warning light on a car. If the "low oil level" light comes on, then you do an oil change. Logical. Would you rather get an axe and smash the warning light? But many do just that: instead of treating a headache first with a refill of magnesium, protein and vitamins, an aspirin is swallowed and the symptom pushed away. That is also exactly what many doctors do. An example: when an overweight patient "with a bright warning light" comes to his practice for high blood pressure, first and foremost the food problem must be solved. The treatment plan should be more antihypertensive potassium and magnesium from fruits and vegetables, weight loss and sports. Due to this blood pressure, blood sugar and blood fats will, in many cases, return to the normal range. Instead, an antihypertensive medication is prescribed, i.e. "the warning light is smashed with an axe." Due to the unchanged poor diet this patient will be back soon with high blood fats. Then a lipid-lowering agent is added. Another warning light shattered. Thus one turns the patient little by little into an expensive drug addict, instead of first reducing the cause – the obesity – or at least prescribing a required participation in a weight-loss and nutrition course. Medicine has degenerated into a costly repair shop due to suboptimal nutrition. 75% of diseases are diet related. The general public has to pay for the bad habits and sloppy nutrition of those who treat their biochemical machine irresponsibly at best, and who do not know when they are driving it into a wall. The "all-inclusive" mentality of patients and a health system that relies on medicines to take care of symptoms rather than focus on prevention and individual responsibility, is a big mistake. It costs us hundreds of billions of dollars. Money wasted on avoidable problems.

Diet is a personal responsibility

Make your 70 billion cells and your metabolism fit, which is what life and health really need: essential vitamins, minerals, trace elements, protein and omega-3 fats from fish. But please do not expect fast miracles: 70% of the cells of your body are replaced completely within 8 to 12 months. Thus they need time to rebuild your body. Food low in nutrients and fatty junk food does not get you into top shape and can only make you heavier.

Reasons for micronutrient deficiencies

Why does a balanced diet no longer cover the minimal requirement of micronutrients?
80% of the participants in my seminars say that they eat well and don't need vitamins. But when I ask for more details, it is amazing what they buy and actually eat. Five studies in three countries with 80,000 people show that today's diet no longer achieves a sufficient amount of micronutrients. Why is that?

There are six factors that are responsible for the decline in micronutrient intake in our diet:

- A change in the composition of the diet. Twice as much fat, especially saturated animal fat and ten times as much sugars as 200 years ago.
- Ice age leached soils in northern Europe and the use of chemicals.
- Food storage and long transportation distances.
- Food processing: cleaning, peeling, boiling, blanching, pasteurisation, preservation, irradiation and microwave heating.
- Changes in eating habits: restaurants, cafes, convenience foods.
- Ignorance and laziness.

These six factors are the reason that in a 1000 calories, only a fraction of the vitamins, minerals and trace elements are contained of what the immune system and the metabolism would have received from 1,000 calories in the early times of evolution. Normally you would rely on your instinct in your search for food. This doesn't really work in a supermarket. Children now like artificial flavours in yogurts even better than a real fruit addition. We must therefore increasingly replace instinct with knowledge. You as a reader of this book belong to the top ten per cent of the population who are interested in nutrition and want to take your health into your own hands.

Deficiency - a consequence of changed food composition

Myth No 1:
"Diets have not fundamentally changed for our metabolism."
Many people don't even seem to know that vitamins and minerals can be found in fruits and vegetables. Accordingly, these foods with their high proportion of micronutrients play a far too minor role in their diet.

What are empty calories?
Too many "empty" calories are eaten. Fats or sugars do not contain micronutrients! Vitamins are needed in order to metabolize these foods at all.

Thus, the empty calories of a sugary or high fat diet are more like "vitamin robbers". Instead of micronutrient-rich foods - fruits, vegetables, and whole grain cereals – needed to fuel the metabolism with organic materials many burden the body mainly with fat and sugar. Diabetes and cardiovascular disease are the most obvious result of this diet.

Have some "fun" and the next time you visit the beach imagine the eating habits of your fellow citizens who are walking by: here is the cream cheese cake-devouring heart attack candidate, closely followed by the early diabetic with a micronutrient deficiency. And there the fat, clogged up fast food type and his three "nutritionally abused" children with their chronically swollen fat cells. The only reason these people are living longer today than in the Stone Age is the use of antibiotics and the fully comprehensive repair medicine. The metabolism and immune system of these people are much less potent than that of their ancestors, the cavemen. How today's diet has changed compared to the Stone Age, you can see in the table below.[127]

	Prehistoric man in the Palaeolithic era	Today
Percentage of **proteins** in the energy supply	20-35%	↓ 10-20%
Percentage of **fats** in the energy supply	20%	↑ 40%
Percentage of **carbohydrates** in the energy supply Of which are simple sugars	40-50% 15-30 g	40-50% ↑ 120-150 g
Fiber	45 g	↓ 20 g

Compared to the Stone Age, we get: half as much protein, twice as much micronutrient-free fat and five times as much vitamin-poor simple sugars.

Sugar and weight gain

The consumption of quick carbohydrates from highly processed and low-fiber foods has increased fivefold. Especially under observation: simple sugars. The metabolism is not adapted

GOOD TO KNOW

Omega-3 fatty acids
The valuable omega-3 fats are barely found in our modern diets. They are so important to our health: they are the vital building blocks of messengers that help to prevent rheumatic inflammation, reduce the risk of diabetes by half, reduce the risk of heart attacks and they are the building blocks of a fit brain.

to such large amounts of quickly available energy. The body must store the superfluous energy with the help of insulin into storage facilities – the fat cells. From there, the energy often comes out only with difficulty. It's like a one-way street into fat cells. Thus the year-rings grow around the belly and now account for every second German being overweight.

By contrast the energy from natural foods - whole grains, fruits and vegetables - is absorbed into the bloodstream much more slowly. This diet also results in a much more consistent level of energy. The highs and lows and the energy holes with sugar cravings go away.

You do not only get fatter from this sugar-rich diet, but your cells receive too few micronutrients. The 70

GOOD TO KNOW

Concentrated organic materials in fresh juices

Fresh juices are important today in addition to frozen foods in order to consume larger amounts of biological substances. With a juicer you can prepare some fresh juice with carrots, celery, beetroot and apples within 5 minutes. Juicing does not cause a loss of vitamins like cooking does. There is no better way to refuel phytochemicals and micronutrients than with fresh juices. The juice guru Dr. Norman Walker, who made orange juice popular in the U.S. in the 50s, drank large quantities of fresh vegetable juices every day. At the age of 116, he has written his last juice book. Tip: Add a little oil to the juice. Many plant substances are 'fat soluble' and can be absorbed by the intestines only with a little fat.

billion cells of obese people are therefore generally refuelled the least with micronutrients.

Double the "killer fats"

The average person receives almost 40% of their calories from fat: sausage, cheese, butter, fatty dairy products like cream, hidden fats in French fries, candy and fast food. Saturated fat - mostly animal fatty dairy (aside from excess calories ideal for the love handles) - contains absolutely nothing that the body can use sensibly. These are "empty fat calories". Prehistoric man also ate a lot of meat. But the fat content of a wild animal is 4 to 5% as opposed to a barn animal that has a fat content of about 30%. Over the course of evolution, there was no food that consisted almost exclusively of fat. Nature has not yet equipped us with the necessary "metabolic software" for flooding the blood with fats. And if you want to burn fat you need vitamin C and other important antioxidants, which prevent the fat from depositing on artery walls. The consequences of fat consumption and antioxidant-deficiencies are diet-related cardiovascular diseases.

Halving the proportion of protein

The intake of protein is decreased nearly by half. This is perhaps new to you, because over and over again it is claimed that we get enough protein. However, muscle growth, the immune system and all cells need lots of protein, which serve as building material, for detoxification and repair processes. You can boost your metabolism and your immune system tremendously if you consume more high-quality protein. The easiest way is with a delicious protein shake. The advantage: there is hardly any fat in a protein concentrate. For it is only the high fat protein sources - like full-fat milk and meat products - that are unhealthy. The protein itself is healthy. Protein also decreases the appetite and stimulates the production of nerve messengers that make you happy, concentrated and content.

The new food pyramid.

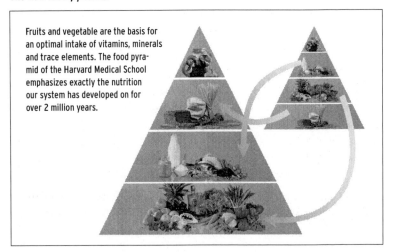

Fruits and vegetable are the basis for an optimal intake of vitamins, minerals and trace elements. The food pyramid of the Harvard Medical School emphasizes exactly the nutrition our system has developed on for over 2 million years.

You get only half the dietary fiber necessary

Fibers have important functions: they clean the intestines and prevent a too rapid influx of energy into the bloodstream. The consequences of a low-fiber diet include: constipation, bacterial overgrowth and intestinal cancer.

The new food pyramid

Over two million years of human history, man was a hunter (high protein content) and a gatherer (high vitamin content of plants). Only 10,000 years ago did man, with the help of agriculture, become sedentary. Since then we eat more carbohydrates from cereal products. Our metabolism is thus well

STUDY: NUTS REDUCE THE RISK OF CARDIOVASCULAR DISEASE

Nuts - Power packs for in between

In-between snacks when you are at work are important. But instead of munching empty calories from candy bars, rather grab some nuts more often. They are a miracle of nature - no other food is packed with as many nutrients: zinc, selenium, vitamins and antioxidant phytochemicals. After all, a whole tree can grow from a small nut. The classic trail mix is the perfect brain food for you to be fit in the workplace. By the way, nuts reduce heart attacks like no other nutrient package could do.

Study participants	Period of time	Result
86,000 women	14 years	↓ 41% lower risk of fatal heart attacks with higher nut consumption[128]
31,208 men and women	6 years	↓ 52% lower risk of fatal heart diseases with higher nut consumption[129]
35,000 women	8 years	↓ 67% lower risk of fatal heart attacks with higher nut consumption[130]

adapted to more protein. Our biochemical factory especially needs more micronutrients, which are now lost since the industrial processing of food. The new food pyramid takes this into consideration and again places fruits and vegetables, i.e. vitamins, minerals and trace elements, as a base. The next step is low-fat protein. The "whole grain" carbohydrates are placed only in the third layer. At the very top of the pyramid we see the micronutrient-poor, highly processed, fast carbohydrates. With this diet you stay slim, you can eat as much as you want and could avoid 70% of the diet-related diseases.

TIP

Your metabolism craves iodine, selenium, zinc and chromium from whole grains, fruits & vegetables and not empty calories. Can't make it 5 times a day? Then an additional multi-mineral product brings the craved trace elements back and makes your metabolism come alive and helps the immune system to become stronger. However: don't combine several products that all have trace elements in them. Trace elements can easily be overdosed.

80% fewer micronutrients

Through the great amount of empty calories from processed carbohydrates and fat, the micronutrient intake is decreased by about 80%! Our metabolism has not been able to adapt to this lack of biological substances. The short term effects are: decreased performance and a weak immune system. In the long term, empty calories are responsible for diet-related diseases.

Make your metabolism strong again. Micronutrient deficiency was yesterday. Recharge your life force through a winning diet filled with vitamins, minerals and micronutrients.

Micronutrient deficiency due to depleted soils and chemicals

Myth No 2:
"Of course we get all the micronutrients we need in a rich country like Germany"
Germany and northern Europe have a shortage of chromium, zinc, iodine and selenium in the soil due to the washout of trace elements during the Ice Age. Consequences of the lack of supply of minerals include:

- Enlargement of the thyroid: the thyroid gland becomes enlarged when there is an iodine deficiency to filter even the last crumbs of iodine from the blood. A goiter is formed. Thus due to iodine deficiency there are 90,000 unnecessary thyroid surgeries and costly prescriptions of thyroid hormones. The costs of these amounts to up to one billion euros per year in Germany.[132] Only a kilometer across the Swiss border, where iodine is added to foods by law, this condition hardly ever occurs. Absurd: Implementation of cost savings is almost entirely unknown in German politics, although it is talked about so often. The iodine-laws of former East Germany were abolished during reunification. After a series of examinations, 20% of the members of the German parliament was shown to have an enlarged thyroid gland...
- Weakening of the immune system: zinc and selenium are essential for the functioning of the immune system and provide building blocks for the production of endogenous antioxidant enzymes.

Optimal selenium intake through food cannot be achieved in Germany

Country	Selenium intake per day
Germany, northern Europe	40-60 µg
USA	60-150 µg
Canada	150-200 µg
Japan	150-200 µg
Optimal Selenium intake	150-200 µg[131]

Another example of the mineral deficiency is the use of insecticides. This can interfere with plants' absorption of minerals, because insecticides kill microorganisms in the small roots, which are required for mineral absorption. The use of certain insecticides may also considerably reduce the vitamin content. For example, the use of propionic acid, an antifungal agent, is to blame for the destruction of 90% of vitamin E in cereal products.

Storage and transport destroy micronutrients

Myth No 3:
"I always eat fresh and thus vitamin rich."
This is what I often hear from my seminar participants. My answer:
- **Yes,** you get a variety of plant materials from fresh fruit and vegetables that can never be pressed into a pill. These plant compounds are effective against cancer and cardiovascular disease. That's why you should eat fruits and vegetables five times a day. Most of these plant compounds are also relatively stable for storage and cooking.
- **No,** you do not get enough vitamins. In fact, vitamins are very easily destroyed, since they are highly sensitive to storage, oxygen, light, heat and all other processing.

Have you ever thought about how much time vegetables and fruits are on a truck when they are transported across a continent? How long they spent in hypermarkets before coming to your supermarket outside refrigerated sections? Then on top of that many people store them at home in a decorative fruit bowl until they finally eat them. What's left in an apple after being shipped from New Zealand? How big is the influence of storage time on vitamin content?

- A freshly harvested, ripe apple contains 10 mg of vitamin C per 100 g. After eleven weeks of storage at 3° C, the apple only contains 5 mg: a loss of 50%.
- Harvested unripe – like the "inter-continental-transport-fruits", for example New Zealand apples, also contain fewer vitamins than ripened fruit.
- Spinach loses 70% of its folate after three days of being stored at room temperature.

GOOD TO KNOW

Health from the freezer
Frozen vegetables are not only convenient, since you can always have them in the house and you do not have to clean them, they are also healthy. Analyses show that frozen vegetables are richer in vitamins than vegetables that are stored even for a short time, because they are frozen immediately after harvest and therefore not stored unrefrigerated for an extended period. Your cells rejoice!

The table clearly shows the loss of micronutrients in spinach.

Temperature-dependent vitamin C loss in spinach due to storage

	After 24 hours	After 48 hours
4 °C	↓ 22%	↓ 34%
12 °C	↓ 26%	↓ 40%
20 °C	↓ 36%	↓ 52%

Fruit does not belong in decorative fruit bowls, but in the refrigerator. The new refrigerators with the Zero-Degree-Zone does not only decrease the loss of vitamins, but also saves a lot of money as fruits and vegetables keep twice as long, thus being thrown out less frequently.

Processing of foods

Myth No 4:
"In preparation and processing of the food very little gets lost."
47 micronutrients are essential for the functioning of our metabolism. 70% of the foods that are consumed today are industrially processed, pasteurized, sterilized, washed, peeled, cooked, refined or irradiated. A large part of the sensitive organic substances is lost. Important health promoting substances are peeled away, destroyed or changed in their chemical structure so that they are no longer bio-available.

Then, additives, colourings, artificial flavors, preservatives, and pH stabilizers are added, which in turn can cause chemical reactions with the nutrients. Many of these new chemical structures can only be disposed of by the organism and are involved in the development of cancer.

Loss of vitamins during processing

This is how "vitamin-rich" your diet really is: spinach loses 80% of folate[133] after cooking it for 2 minutes. When blanching frozen vegetables, 95% of vitamin C, 60% of vitamin B_1 and 40% of vitamin B_2 are lost.[135] In the tables next page the vitamin losses are calculated in the production of flour.

> **TIP**
>
> Eat more whole wheat products, from which the important micronutrients and minerals have not been removed.

Vitamin loss in the production of white flour[134]

	Whole grain	Refined flour	Loss
Carotene	0.23 mg	0.06 mg	↓ 74%
Vitamin B$_1$	0.48 mg	0.06 mg	↓ 88%
Vitamin B$_2$	0.14 mg	0.03 mg	↓ 79%
Vitamin B$_3$	5.10 mg	0.70 mg	↓ 86%
Pantothenic acid	1.18 mg	0.21 mg	↓ 82%
Vitamin B$_6$	0.44 mg	0.18 mg	↓ 59%

Loss of minerals and micronutrients through processing

Industrial processing leads to significant mineral and micronutrient losses. What is left?

- Compared to brown rice, polished rice has only 25% of copper, manganese and chromium.
- White flour contains only 7 µg of zinc compared to 134 µg in whole wheat flour. The valuable micronutrient-rich surface layers of the grain on the other hand go into animal feed. The farmer knows what his cattle needs the most.

An optimal metabolism and a powerful immune system can hardly be achieved with our modern diet. The four trace elements manganese, zinc, selenium and copper are for example part of the important endogenous antioxidant enzymes that neutralize free radicals. A lack of manganese, zinc and selenium also causes an accumulation of heavy metals in the body. These trace elements detoxify your body as they bind to heavy metals.

All minerals, trace elements and vitamins are part of all important metabolic reactions. Deficiencies in these essential micronutrients cause a rapid increase in diet-related diseases.

Loss of minerals during the production of white flour[136]

Manganese	↓ 86%
Zinc	↓ 78%
Selenium	↓ 70%
Copper	↓ 68%
Iron	↓ 76%
Cobalt	↓ 89%
Molybdenum	↓ 48%
Chromium	↓ 40%
Magnesium	↓ 85%
Potassium	↓ 77%
Phosphor	↓ 71%
Calcium	↓ 60%

Loss of micronutrients and changed eating habits

Those who have a job don't have much time to look for something to eat during the lunch break. It is difficult to find something edible of high quality. Often there is no other option than to eat at fast food restaurants, university, hospitals, nursing homes or corporate cafeterias. What do these foods have left after they have already been cooked and kept warm?

Here a few examples of vitamin-loss:
- Salad bar: chopped salad and shredded vegetables lose 30% of their vitamins per hour due to their contact with oxygen and light.
- A cut up tomato loses 50% of the important antioxidant lycopene per hour.
- A study of hospital food in England showed: 100 g of peas during thawing had 20.5 mg vitamin C, 8.1 mg after cooking, after an hour in the food trolley 3.7 mg, and 1.1 mg when they arrived on the plate of the patients.[137]

A study on quality assurance in a hospital in Freiburg, Germany showed that the micro-nutrient content of food was barely sufficient to avoid the main deficiencies.[138] How then should a patient be healthy and get better? B-vitamins are involved in the rebuilding of all cells. Vitamin C alone is part of 15,000 metabolic reactions - including wound repair. Most patients that are discharged need to be nursed at home again only to compensate for nutrient deficiencies. In business cafeterias, snack bars and buffet restaurants the loss of micronutrients is similar. With such a micronutrient-poor meal in the afternoon you can barely perform. That would require more protein and vitamins and as little fat as possible.

Logistics is important

Bring your own fruits and nuts for in between, rather than the fatty chocolate bars, the sugary sweets or the chips from the machine. When the fruit is sitting on your desk, it will also be eaten. The more frequently you eat outside the home, the more important it is to at least eat healthy food at home. One thing is clear: if you consume 1,000 calories of "micronutrient poor" food per day, then on the following evening or on weekends you cannot catch up by eating regular food. With additional vitamins you can achieve at least the minimum intake.

"Lucy" – Micronutrient intake 10,000 years ago and today

What would have been found in the soup bowl of the Stone Age woman Lucy? The two-time Nobel laureate Linus Pauling has calculated the micronutrient content of the diet of "Lucy", our ancestor three million years ago. Based on 2,500 calories, "Lucy" would have consumed 3 times the amount of micronutrients as recommended by the German Society for Nutrition. For vitamin C, this was calculated at 40 times their recommended intake (RDA).

Changed eating habits, depleted soils, storage, transportation and industrial processing cause the micronutrient to contain per 1,000 calories only a fraction of the amounts necessary for the optimal functioning of the organism. The variety in the supermarkets overshadows the fact that the most highly processed foods, for reasons of durability, are harvested while unripe and stored for long periods of time. It is unrealistic to assume that working people in modern industrial society can always eat freshly harvested, well refrigerated and optimally prepared foods. Nevertheless, most people believe that they have all the nutrients, to provide an optimal metabolism and immune system to perform at high level.

The myth of the varied diet

Can you achieve the minimum intake of all micronutrients through a varied diet?
Overflowing shelves in supermarkets create the impression of abundance, which upon closer analysis of food turns out to be a bubble. Due to the loss of micronutrients in current foods it is difficult to achieve the minimum values with a "varied diet". This leads to the paradoxical situation of a "deficiency in abundance".

A French and Dutch study debunk the myth of the "varied diet". Their analysis shows that with less than 2,500 calories, only 80% of the recommended, already low values, can be achieved.[139, 140] On a daily basis modern woman consumes usually only 1,850 calories. A higher caloric intake, even with a "more varied diet", is not desirable for women for reasons of weight gain.

> **GOOD TO KNOW**
>
> **A varied diet – is that enough?**
> The optimal intake of micronutrients is about three times higher than the minimum RDAs. However, according to recent analysis, 2500 calories of a balanced diet contain only 80% of these minimum requirements. The rest should be supplemented.

Daily allowance – completely outdated

First of all, for all American readers: I will be using the German RDA values instead of U.S. RDA values. It doesn't make much of a difference if the two rating systems vary by a couple of milligrams for one or the other vitamin. Generally the notion that you can calculate a daily allowance for trillions of metabolic reactions where vitamins are needed is absurd anyway. The best scientists can do is research what humans ate during the time of evolution. This is the optimal level. And, even though most American readers are not used to reading anything other than works by American authors, it's easy enough to transfer the general idea to your own life.

It's very interesting to think about how RDA values come about at all. The German RDA defines a minimum requirement that has little to do with optimal health care. If you look closer at the intake recommendations, you will notice the following problems:

- The recommended intakes for various states for certain vitamins differ by up to 20-fold![141] Instead of scientific research, political viability determines the national intake recommendations.
- The definition of vitamin deficiency is out-dated, because the guidelines were developed on the basis of knowledge about vitamins from the 50s and 60s of the last century.
- The long-term consequences of vitamin deficiency and the prevention of diseases caused by free radical antioxidants have not been taken into consideration.
- Even within the German Nutrition Society (DGE) there are different schools of thought. The DGE only makes a decision if it is unanimous. That is why nothing changes in daily vitamin allowance as long as there is even one vote against it.

Ups and Downs – how politics are connected to the daily allowance recommendations

Why are the government's policies and recommended intake levels not the optimal values for prevention?

Folate for example reveals the absurdity of the official recommended intakes very clearly. An average of 90% of the population has a folate deficiency. Nine out of ten readers of this book have too little of this vitamin. However, folate is essential for your health.

It is worthwhile to treat folate in more detail. Folate is the diva - the most sensitive - among the vitamins. During three days of storage at supermarket temperatures 70% of folate is lost, another 80% of the remaining folate is lost during two minutes of cooking. However, our genetic conditions, i.e. our metabolic software, have not changed since the invention of the refrigerator and stove. The minimal allowance values do not represent an optimal intake. An optimal supply may be around 3x the RDA as it was during the time of evolution.

State regulations: The crime of folic acid

Victim No 1: Pregnant women

How does a folate-deficiency affect pregnant women?

Folate deficiency affects women of childbearing age severely. According to the German National Nutrition Survey, 99% of women between 19 and 35 years of age get too little folate.[142] Especially women who take the pill (contraceptive), have extreme folate deficiency, as the pill, like many drugs, blocks folate absorption in the body. Folate deficiency increases the risk of giving birth to children with a malformation (the neural tube defect) by 70%. Each year there are 1,400 neural tube defects in Germany, which can result in either abortion or disability. An additional 800 mcg folic acid daily can reduce this risk accordingly by up to 70%. For 35 years this has been confirmed by extensive studies.

In 1989, during the budget crisis in the U.S.A., despite the results of these studies, the folate recommendation was halved from 400 µg to 200 µg. The depressing reason: the higher the recommended standards are, the more expensive the social budget gets. This is because the U.S. issued food stamps for welfare and they had to comply with the RDA. In those years this sadly resulted in the birth of thousands of disabled children.

As recently as 1992 the FDA, the Food and Drug Administration, confiscated vitamin tablets which contained a statement on the package that folic acid during and before pregnancy dramatically reduces the risk of malformations in infants.

As early as in 1993 the public pressure became so great that the FDA had to change their attitude. In the Journal of the American Medical Association, the FDA all of a sudden rejoiced that the relationship between folate deficiency and malformations was "one of the most exciting research results at the end of this century". The results of large studies had already been known for 20 years! The value was once again set to 400 µg.

In 1997, five years later, the German Nutrition Society (DGE) finally took a position and admitted that at least those women planning to become pregnant should take an additional 400 µg of folic acid, because the recommended value cannot be achieved by diet alone.[143]

Victim No 2: Patients with heart attacks

Heart attacks due to a folate deficiency are common!

Since 1998 folic acid has to be added to basic foods in the U.S. The reason: 50,000 heart attacks in the U.S. are caused solely due to a folate deficiency. Prof. Pietrzik calculates 15,000 corresponding cases for Germany. Since folate deficiency greatly increases the risk of cardiovascular disease, it is only logical that with the additional administration of this vitamin, money can be saved in the national health budget. This way research is wisely chaneled into prevention in the United States.

In 2000, the DGE also increased the tentative recommendation for all adults from 300 µg to 400 µg. This, according to DGE, could of course be achieved with a wholesome diet. Since 90% of the population does not even achieve 300 mcg this demonstrates the fact of the absurd misinformation from national nutrition societies which misleads the consumer.

Seven years later, in 2007, the DGE called a press conference "folate - the forgotten vitamin". Now the experts were cheering that one must enrich flour to correct the folate deficiency. It is emphasized however that vitamin pills cannot solve the problem. Unfortunately, this legal enrichment is politically not feasible. At the speed of German politics, it will probably take another 10 years or 14,000 malformative births and 155,000 deaths from cardiovascular disease until there is a statutory regulation regarding folic acid fortification.

> **GOOD TO KNOW**
>
> **The rate of intake recommendations**
> As with stock prices, the recommended intake levels go up and down. A real analysis of the fundamentals of new metabolic and clinical studies in is lacking most cases. Depending on the political "feasibility" micronutrients can also be noted as "low". However, the "micronutrient ratings" are rising in many countries because lately the health care departments have recognized the potential savings.

My advice:

Until then, we can confidently take vitamin pills with folic acid and reduce the risk for cardiovascular disease, cancer and dementia ourselves. When you look at these arbitrary changes you can clearly see how the supply is halved despite recommendations of existing research results and a few years later, when it seems opportune, it is again doubled. Then suddenly, even basic foods are fortified with it. Some countries, however, even sleep through these measures. Similarly confusing are the recommendations for other vitamins, for example for vitamin E

and vitamin C. The differences between what is good enough for an American or a European vary all the time. Let alone what is good enough for someone from the third world.

Admitting that 99% of inhabitants in the Western world do not reach the recommended folate intake, one should question the usefulness of RDA values altogether. The nutrition societies want to show that you can get everything you need with a good diet. Indeed, 1% of the population does in the case of folate. This is absurd.

Outdated ideas about vitamin deficiency

The reason for the RDA values is the prevention of deficiency diseases that are caused by vitamin deficiency. These include, for example, scurvy (formerly known as a sailor's disease), vitamin C deficiency, anemia through folate and vitamin B_{12} deficiency, rickets in children with vitamin D deficiency and Beriberi due to vitamin-B1 deficiency. To protect against these serious diseases, a minimum of vitamins is necessary. Of course, today in the Western world nobody dies of these diseases anymore. The current problems and cost drivers in health care lie in cardiovascular disease, cancer, osteoporosis and dementia.

As a rule of thumb, the absolute minimum intake recommendations were increased a little bit, in order to get a value for the daily recommended allowance of vitamins and minerals. It is of course nonsense that one could accurately calculate in exact milligrams the necessary intake of vitamins for the trillions of metabolic reactions. It is just as absurd as to take the same values for all people between the ages of 18 and 65 with different dietary and life-style habits.

With other vitamins, which in the case of a deficit do not immediately show the consequences of deficiency symptoms or diseases until many years later, for example with cardiovascular disease due to vitamin D deficiency or the cell damage caused by antioxidant deficiency, the recommendation is even more approximate.

The benchmark in the U.S. of 12 mg of vitamin E per day was created by calculating how much vitamin E was in the soup bowl of the average American in the 50s who showed no major signs of deficits. However, a long-term consequence of a vitamin E deficiency is a greatly increased risk for cardiovascular disease and cancer.

Therefore, new reference values are necessary for consumers today. Minimum intake values are misleading. The basis for calculating the RDA should not be the short-term, but rather the long-term effects of a vitamin deficiency; this must be brought into focus. The experience of long-term clinical trials can provide good clues for that.

The six stages of micronutrient deficiency

Stage 1 and 2: Depletion of tissue and bone content

Why do you hardly notice a micronutrient deficiency?
Blood tests for micronutrients outside of the cells very often show completely normal results. The reason is that a lack of intake first manifests itself in cell and tissue content of micronutrients within the cells. Here are some examples:

- The white blood cells that normally store 40-times the vitamin C content, contain less and less vitamin C. Thus, the immune system loses strength. You become susceptible to infections. The blood test measures the vitamin content on the outside of the immune cells.
- The magnesium content in the blood is normal, although the content decreases within the cells. This slows down the metabolism in the cell.
- The content of vitamin E in the blood (outside of the cell) is normal, although there is less of this vitamin in the cell membranes. Thus, the cell membranes become more and more damaged by free radicals.
- The calcium content in the blood is normal, although within the bones, a loss of bone density due to a lack of calcium is shown.

Thus it always comes down to the measurement method. In stages 1 and 2, vitamin blood tests often do not show the full picture. At this stage a blood test for oxidative stress caused by free radicals (see page 25) can be more valuable to indicate if there is an insufficient supply of antioxidants such as vitamins C and E.

Stages 3 and 4: Deficiency symptoms – slowed-down metabolism and an accumulation of damage

The micronutrient blood levels are normal. You are, however, mostly in the lower third of the norm.

Since the tissue stores are depleted, more and more metabolic processes as well as the production of hormones are placed on the backburner and regulated down. How can we feel this? Maybe your performance has decreased and concentration and memory diminished. Often we are more prone to stress and suffer from mood swings.

Why is the lower third of the normal range of vitamins in the blood not enough?

Let me give you some examples of deficiency sypmtoms that may occur then: Women more often suffer from premenstrual syndrome. The fat burning does not work perfectly, and you are more prone to infection. In stages 3 and 4, which can last 15 to 30 years, the foundations of the degenerative diseases of the cardiovascular system, nervous system (Parkinson's disease, Alzheimer's disease or senile dementia) and for cancer are built. Failing antioxidant levels can first be measured by the initial membrane damage to the cells. The body cells age prematurely due to the genetic and metabolic changes that accumulate.

The micronutrient deficiency at this stage can only be recognized by minor symptoms, to which initially no attention is paid. Which symptoms are a sign of a micronutrient deficiency, can be found on page 95. It is always suspicious when you suffer from several well-known and typical deficiency symptoms of a particular micronutrient.

What you can do now

In these stages, you can correct it through a change of diet with five servings of fruits and vegetables daily, more whole grain products and additional micronutrients, because the damage has not yet translated into lasting diseases. This optimizes your blood values. After a few months the cells have been replaced and will function better, and you will also notice a difference in your metabolism. On these levels, micronutrients can act in these stages:

1. Optimization of the metabolism to increase performance.
2. Supporting the immune system to fight infection.
3. Long-term protection of health.

If you raise your blood levels, the goal should always be to bring these up to the upper third of the normal range, because the standard values are mean values or average values for the entire population. Consider the average diet of the population. You only need to look in the shopping cart of the person in front of you in the supermarket queue. To be in the middle of this average blood value is certainly no great feat, and certainly not the best for your health and performance. With vitamins, minerals and micronutrients, you could "tune" your blood levels in this upper third level. Also important is a test for an elevated homocysteine, to determine a too low intake of folate, B_{12} and B_6 for your metabolism.

Stage 5: Functional disorders – symptoms that require treatment

What can you expect from micronutrients in stage 5?

At this stage symptoms need to be treated and you suffer from the typical manifestations of chronic micronutrient deficiency: depression, chronic fatigue syndrome, burn-out, high blood pressure, high blood fat levels, high blood sugar, precursors of malignant cells.

INFO

Micronutrients are effective primarily for the prevention of diseases. Although the therapeutic use of micronutrients activates self-healing powers, you should not have unrealistic expectations.

What micronutrients can do now

At this stage many people have completely unrealistic expectations of vitamins. You want to quickly adjust the balance that has resulted from decades of neglect. Micronutrients work mainly in prevention. Therefore, we cannot consider micronutrients as medicine for repairing gene and cell damage or a completely derailed metabolism.

By administering targeted and high dosed micronutrients the metabolism may be affected and enzymatic repair processes set in motion. This is a therapeutic use of micronutrients, which definitely belongs in the hands of an experienced orthomolecular doctor! This is neither a task for the typical American 1,000 page self-help guides of the "self-pharmacy" type nor the task of an employee of a health food shop who works in his own interest. A list of orthomolecular specialists can be found through an Internet search engine.

Stage 6: Pathological disorders – irreversible damage

The changes to genes, cells, damage to organs and free radical diseases such as cancer, heart attacks, diabetes and cataracts that accumulated over time cannot be reversed.

What possibilities are left at this stage?

Orthomolecular therapy, meaning taking high doses of micronutrients, can only accompany traditional medicine. In cancer, for example, the free radicals, which are increased in radiation therapy, can be intercepted, so that healthy tissue is spared and in cardiovascular disease the risk of a second heart attack may be reduced. The actual damage cannot be reversed, rather only delayed.

INFO

At stage 6 the real damage can no longer be reversed by micronutrients, only delayed.

The six stages of micronutrient deficiency

Stage	1–2 Deficient intake	3–4 Deficiency symptoms	5 Functional disturbances	6 Pathological disturbances
Consequences	↓ depletion of micronutrient tissue content	↓ metabolism, ↓ degenerative damages to cells, ↓ immune deficiency	↓ symptoms requiring treatment	↓ irreversible damages
↓ stored and intracellular micronutrients	decrease			
↓ micro-nutrient blood levels		decrease		
↓ activity of vitamin-dependent enzymes and hormones		decrease		
↓ disturbances in the metabolism ↓ degenerative damage		increase		

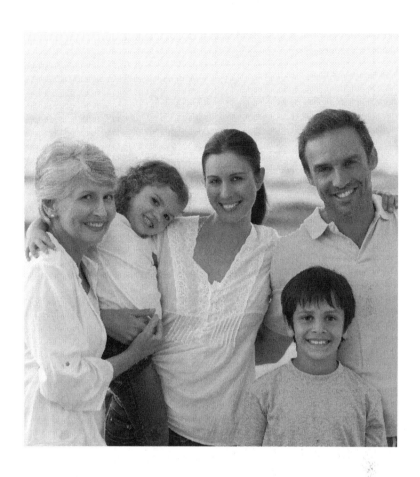

CHAPTER 5

Who Needs Micronutrients?

Why should you be in the upper third of the vitamin blood levels? What do blood levels of champions look like? Why is the minimum intake too little? What is a safe intake? Why do young women, the elderly, smokers, athletes, people exposed to contaminants, diabetics and many other groups need more micronutrients? How do micronutrients help to detoxify?

Tune up your blood levels

When you measure your micronutrients' blood levels, it is important to be able to interpret the results. The standard values vary from state to state, depending on how the average population is supplied with micronutrients.

A good example is selenium: as Germany is a selenium-deficient area; the average standard value for the German population is specified as a low 70 µg/l. With this much too low value "you are in the normal range". However, the World Health Organization (WHO) sets the average at 200 µg/l.

INFO

When you measure your micronutrients' blood levels, it is important to be able to interpret the results. The standard values vary from state to state, depending on how the average population is supplied with micronutrients.

The blood levels of champions

For athletes, it has been done for a long time. Blood levels are optimized to the upper third of the norm, in order to provide optimum performance. But you are a high-performance athlete in many respects - you need nerves of steel at work or in the family and every day you must provide high performance at work. Your performance and your health are your assets and your competitive advantage. By raising the levels of micronutrients in the blood, the metabolism can be optimized. In addition, the nervous system is strengthened, and sick time can be reduced by supporting the immune system. This is also how animals do it in the wild, searching for the freshest food.

What values guarantee optimal performance?

Standard values are often very vague and set low. Optimal values were developed by Dr. Strunz for the famous Forever Young Program in Germany. For better performance and protection you can tune your blood levels in this upper range.

The blood levels of Champions

Micronutrients in the serum	Optimal values	Some advantages
Calcium	> 2,5 mmol/l	Bone protection, better nervous system
Your level		
Magnesium	> 0,9 mmol/l	Lower blood pressure and good nerves
Your level		
Iron Men	1,1-1,5 mg/l	Good oxygen transport to the blood
Women	1,0-1,43 mg/l	Remark: few people need extra iron. Mostly women up to menopause. Only take iron supplements when a doctor prescribes them. Men are almost never iron deficient.
Your level		
Selenium	150-170 µg/l	Cell protection, cancer prevention
Your level		
Folate	25 µg/l	Reduced risk of cardiovascular disease, cancer, dementia
Your level		
Vitamin E	30 µg/ml	Cell protection, decreased risk of cardiovascular diseases
Your level		
Vitamin C	20-30 mg/l	Cell protection, decreased risk of cardiovascular diseases
Your level		
Vitamin D*	30-60 µg/ml	Bone protection, reduced risk of cancer
Vitamin D**	60-120 µg/ml	Bone protection, reduced risk of cancer
Your level		
Vitamin B_1	40-100 µg/ml	Good nerves
Your level		
Vitamin B_2	150-250 µg/ml	Energy metabolism
Your level		
Vitamin B_6	100-200 µg/ml	Fast cell build-up
Your level		
Vitamin B_{12}	500-1000 µg/ml	Psychological stability in old age, reduced risk of dementia
Your level		

* 25-Hydroxycholecalciferol
** 1,25 Dihydroxycholecalciferol
What other functions vitamins, minerals and micronutrients influence can be found on page 145.

The prevention of deficiency symptoms is not enough

"100 ml of this juice can cover 60% of the RDA requirement for vitamin C." You already know what to think of such information. The RDA-values are far too low.

The consumers believe in the RDAs and think they have done the best for themselves. But what do these values not take into consideration?

- Optimal performance is directly related to an above average micronutrient intake.
- A powerful immune system is dependent on an optimum supply of micronutrients.
- Long-term protection against free radicals is directly related to an increased intake of antioxidants.
- Lifestyle habits, genetic conditions and already existing diseases can multiply the demand. Therefore you cannot set an average requirement for all people.
- Detoxification mechanisms, that are increasingly active in disposing increased quantities of pollutants, result in a much greater demand for certain micronutrients.

The intake recommendations speculate on how many milligrams of micronutrients you are entitled to. This chapter should give you a feel for how much micronutrients would really be optimal for your health care.

How much vitamin C do you need?

The optimal intake of vitamin C for the immune system is only achieved when the policemen of the immune system - the lymphocytes and leukocytes - are saturated. During periods of infection the demand of these immune cells can increase tenfold. Without problems, during periods where there are no infections, the leukocytes can store significantly more vitamin C than the RDA.

It is sometimes claimed that a higher intake of vitamin C is 100% eliminated ("expensive urine"). This is not true. Only a portion of vitamin C is excreted. The rest is stored in the cells of the immune system and in various highly sensitive organs such as the retina of your eyes. There, it protects the sensitive cells from oxidative destruction.

In a summary of studies that were made between 1942 and 1982, it is shown that the important immune cells are filled further with vitamin C up to a dose of 1,000 mg.[144]

Also the vitamin C that is excreted has an important function: it binds pollutants, and these are then excreted in the urine.

The more vitamin C is used up because of personal circumstances such as stress, smoking, or is used up to fight infections, the less is excreted. So you need a safety buffer for the different situations/habits/pollutants which you are exposed to. Animals respond flexibly: they simply use sugar to produce vitamin C when they need it. Humans have lost this capacity.

For example, a cigarette needs 30 mg of vitamin C, almost a third of the German RDA of 100 mg. The "trace of vitamin C" of 100 mg may save you from scurvy, but not from an infection that you pick up in the subway, when many people have colds.

How many antioxidants do you need for long-term protection?

Certain organs store antioxidant vitamins to protect themselves. The recommended German RDA doses of 100 mg vitamin C and 14 mg vitamin E does not reduce the cancer rate, nor the number of cardiovascular diseases, nor can the frequency of cataract cases be decreased.

To prevent free radical disease, you must bind the free radicals efficiently. Free radicals are found everywhere, where oxygen is transported (lungs, bloodstream), UV light occurs (skin, eyes), pollution of the environment, medication (liver), or where pollutants accumulate (lungs in smokers) and where the immune system is active (infection, cancer, inflammation, diabetes).

Life expectancy and antioxidants

A low incidence rate of cancer and heart attack may translate into a prolonged life expectancy. An example was a study done with 11,348 Americans. Those receiving 800 mg vitamin C per day as a supplement, compared to those who received only 50 mg, reduced their mortality rate by 35% in the same period and had an extended life expectancy of five years![145] These results are actually not really surprising. Evolution has selected the antioxidant protection system so that in the metabolism it neutralizes the resulting free radicals in the immune system. If the antioxidant vitamins are not supplied in sufficient quantities, the cells and the genetic material will degenerate much sooner. Above all, the damage done to genetic material- the metabolic software of the cell - leads to higher variations in metabolism, resulting in diseases and malfunctions. We age. The early aging process thus leads to a shorter life expectancy.

How much vitamin B do you need?

One thing is certain: you will not achieve 800 mg of folate from a typical Western diet. In the upper third of folate intake, you are best protected from stroke, various forms of cancer and dementia. The better vitamin B refueling may uncover enormous performance reserves and keep your brain fit.

You will have noticed by now that many scientists refuse to accept the minimal RDAs. Instead, they recommend a "safe intake". A possible excess of water soluble vitamins is easily excreted. However, depending on life circumstances, genetics, age and dietary habits, most of it is used up. In the following part I will show you why different target groups need more vitamins.

INFO

B-vitamins are easily excreted, if you do not use them up. Supplementing the minimum RDA with a multivitamin could already improve your metabolism.

"Risk groups" - who needs more micro-nutrients?

Actually, you know it already: you are unique. With your unique genetic material, metabolism, your own lifestyle, your food preferences and health problems.

Amazingly, many people are categorized as a "standard metabolic average citizen" in the calculation of the vitamin intake. People, who due to lifestyle or existing diseases have an increased need, are called "risk groups". A closer look reveals that 80% of the German population can be described as "risk group". You will certainly find yourself belonging to several of these groups outlined in the table. For some of these groups, I will show why the demand is multiplied. The national nutrition societies explicitly spell out these risk groups – be it in small print – who have an increased requirement of micronutrients. However, the large proportion of the population in the small print is quite amazing.

"Risk groups" with an increased need for micronutrients

Without underlying existing disease	Risk factor	People with an underlying existing disease	Risk
During acute Infection	++++	Infarction/Stroke	++++
Smokers	++++	High blood fat levels	++++
Alcohol consumers	++++	Diabetes	++++
Severely stressed	++	High blood pressure	++
Leisure athletes	++	Rheumatism	++
Sunbathers	++	Diseases of the eyes	
Dieting	++	Cataracts, Macular degeneration	++++
Strict vegetarians	+	Precursors of cancer/tumors	++++
Exposed to higher pollutant load	++	High medicine consumption	++
With amalgam fillings	+++	Asthma	+++
The elderly	+++	Allergies	+++
The young	++		
During pregnancy	++++		
Women who take birth control pills	+++		

Smoke pollutants consume antioxidants

With every hit of a cigarette you breathe in approximately 10^{15} (1,000,000,000,000,000) free radicals.[146] Through a chain reaction, these free radicals stimulate other free radicals when they are not neutralized by antioxidants. A cigarette can consume up to 30 mg of vitamin C. A large portion of the available vitamin C is mobilized to the lungs, where the pollutants are directly neutralized. The vitamin C content in smokers can decrease by 40% in the blood and in the leukocytes of the immune system. The consequences of antioxidant deficiency are:

- The upper respiratory system of smokers is vulnerable, because bacteria and viruses are destroyed by a slow and depressed immune system.
- An excess of free radicals leads to abnormal cells in the respiratory system which are not eliminated by the immune system.
- The resulting increased antioxidant deficiency in the bloodstream means that cholesterol is oxidized by free radicals (turns rancid), and sticks more easily to the artery walls. This leads to an eightfold higher risk for cardiovascular disease in smokers.

Passive smokers also inhale many of these pollutants. Thus, vitamin C, as shown by recent studies, is also used up in larger quantities in passive smokers.

The beta-carotene issue

Smokers should not take synthetic beta-carotene till this issue has been cleared up. And right now things are confusing. In one study beta-carotene increased the risk of cancer. This study was completly misrepresented by the tabloid press. For former smokers, beta-carotene reduced the risk of cancer by

STUDIES ON LUNG CANCER

Tip for smokers

Lung cancer is the most common cancer in men and the fifth-most common in women. Eat plenty of fruits and vegetables: In 8 out of 9 trials fruit, and in 12 of 20 trials vegetables, lowered the risk of lung cancer.[147] Lycopene from tomatoes is a potent catcher of free radicals and reduces the risk especially well.[148] Vitamin C decreased lung cancer risk by 34%-37% in several studies involving 68,347 participants.[149, 150]

Smoking also reduces the B-vitamins. That's probably why a high folate intake lowered the risk of lung cancer by 47% in studies with smokers. Folate is responsible for repair mechanisms at the genetic level.[151]

500 mg-1,000 mg vitamin C and a multivitamin tablet with all the B-vitamins should belong to the basic program for smokers.

20%! In smokers who also drank alcohol, the risk of cancer, however, increased under beta-carotene. But it is also known that alcohol strongly increases the risk of lung cancer. Still other important studies, like a Harvard study with 22,000 participants, which lasted over 12 years, have convincingly shown that there is no increased risk for smokers.[152]

In non-smokers beta-carotene in no way increases the risk of getting cancer! Over 100 studies demonstrated a reduction in cancer risk at high beta-carotene levels. But fruits and vegetables are much more potent, because apart from beta-carotene, a whole network of antioxidant plant substances defends the cells. You need this whole antioxidant network.

How do micronutrients dispose of cigarette pollutants?
The need for micronutrients such as zinc and selenium is also increased for the disposal of various heavy metals and other pollutants from cigarette smoke. Intake therefore should be higher. Smokers for example have twice the cadmium levels as non-smokers. With a sufficient supply of zinc, cadmium is discharged from the body.

Alcohol consumes micronutrients

Why do alcohol users have a higher risk for heart attacks?
You like to drink a glass of wine in the evening? Up to 2 glasses of wine reduce the risk for cardiovascular disease, because, like aspirin, alcohol thins the blood. On the other hand, alcohol increases the risk of various cancers, particularly breast, colon and liver cancer and cancers of the upper digestive organs. Alcohol blocks among other things the absorption and the metabolism of folic acid and vitamin B_1 and B_6. Thus a deficiency is created. The B-vitamins, for example, are involved in the repair of damaged DNA. And here the numbers, as always, give a brief overview in order to convince you to take at least additional B-vitamins if you regularly lift up a pint. Breast and colorectal cancers account for 44% of cancer diagnoses in women. In men, colorectal cancer represents a quarter of cancer diagnoses (see studies next page).

Vitamin B_1 for a clear head
To degrade alcohol various micronutrients are also used. This increases your personal needs considerably. Vitamin B_1 is required for the biochemical degradation of alcohol. After a night of drinking, the vitamin B_1 deficiency usually shows itself in the form of a slight memory loss. You may not remember everything. This is because vitamin B_1 along with acetylcholine, is involved in

writing information into memory. Now, if all the B_1-vitamins are blocked by the degradation of alcohol, this information storage will temporarily not work.

B-vitamins significantly reduce the risk of cancer due to alcohol consumption

Study participants	Time frame	Result
32,826 women	13 years	↓ 89% decreased risk of breast cancer in women who drink alcohol daily, but have higher folic acid intake[153]
61,433 women	15 years	↓ 72% decreased risk for intestinal cancer in women who drink alcohol daily, but who have the highest Vitamin B_6 intake[154]
47,931 men	6 years	Triple risk of intestinal cancer in men who drink alcohol daily. ↓ No increased risk in men who drink alcohol daily but who have the highest folic acid intake.[155]

Birth control pills prevent more than just ovulation

The pill reduces the absorption of the following vitamins: B_1, B_2, B_6, folate, B_{12} and E.[156] The absorption of zinc and magnesium is also hindered.[157] In many countries it is considered medical malpractice if folic acid is not prescribed with the pill. Since malformations of the embryo happen in the first 4 weeks of pregnancy it is often too late to add

> **TIP**
>
> The World Health Organization recommends that women who use birth control pills, take additional folic acid.

folate at this stage if you become pregnant because you forgot to take the pill.

Sunbathers need beta-carotene

Increased UV radiation over a longer period of time leads to increased exposure of the skin to free radicals and thus a significant decrease of the radical scavenger beta-carotene in the blood.[158] The decrease in beta-carotene levels runs parallel with the duration of sun exposure.

> **TIP**
>
> With frequent sunbathing on holiday beta-carotene should be taken to protect the skin. Beta-carotene is stored mainly in the skin tissue.

Fit and active when you get older

Older people absorb fewer vitamins. Reasons for this are a decreased food intake and less effective food digestion due to the reduced production of digestive enzymes. Also, nutrients are absorbed much less in the intestines of the elderly.

The third stage of life and the immune system

How do vitamin blood levels differ in healthy and sick elderly people?

The Bethany-study shows how strongly a vitamin deficiency affects health. Here the vitamin status of 50 healthy 75-year-old women (gray bars) was compared to 300 sick seniors (black bars) (see illustration). The result: vitamin deficiency is linked to a depressed immune system.

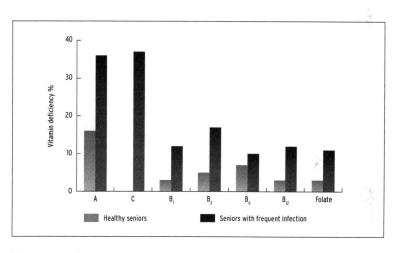

Vitamins support the immune system. Seniors with low vitamin blood levels are sick more often.

The third stage of life and mental performance

How can you increase your mental performance in old age?

The Bethany-study and other research studies[159] also show how much mental performance depends on optimal micronutrient intake. It can be determined that a reduced mental capacity is significantly more common in vitamin deficiencient seniors (gray columns, see illustration). Instead of worrying about a slower mental capacity, you should "refuel" more often with micronutrients of the B-vitamin group.

Depression in the elderly

Older people are often admitted to nursing homes because of appearing mentally unstable conspicuous, depressed or supposedly senile. The poor mental health is often based on a micronutrient deficiency and can be solved by targeting additional intake of micronutrients. Instead, psychotropic drugs are used much too quickly instead of looking to see if there are any nutrient deficiencies that may be the underlying cause. These drugs block micronutrients additionally. Frequent depression and a diminished mental capacity are closely linked to the unavailability of vitamin B_{12} and folate.

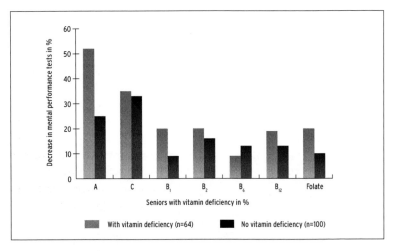

Seniors with and without vitamin deficiency. Micronutrients keep the brain metabolism fit. In the elderly, mental performance increases with a good supply of vitamins (black bars).

Vitamin B_{12} for the immune system, nerves and blood

Older people often have a vitamin B_{12} deficiency[160], young people almost never. To counteract this, i.e. to compensate for the defective function of the transport protein (intrinsic factor), vitamin B_{12} is dosed so highly that a small but sufficient portion passively gets through the intestines into the bloodstream. With a daily additional 500 μg to 1000 μg of vitamin B_{12} as a vitamin pill you could easily correct a vitamin B_{12} deficiency in the elderly. By the way: according to recent studies, high-dose vitamin B_{12} pills work as well as injections by a doctor. 91% of physicians still believe that injections are better, and that makes an expensive visit to the doctor necessary every time.

The depressed often have a Vitamin B$_{12}$ deficiency

Study participants	Result
700 women, over 65 years old	↑ double the risk of depression in women with the lowest Vitamin B$_{12}$ blood levels[161]
694 participants, average age 72. Case control study: comparing participants without depression to participants with depression.	↑ 70% increased risk for depression in participants with the lowest Vitamin B$_{12}$ blood levels[162]

A micronutrient program for the elderly

In elderly people, vitamin deficiency manifests itself in a particularly serious manner, because infections due to immunodeficiency, bone fractures, anemia and loss of mental capacity can quickly lead to a loss of independence and quality of life. Due to a lower yield from food in total, fewer vitamins are absorbed, resulting in a severe vitamin deficiency. In addition the food budget of nursing homes is often only 5 to 6 euros per day per person. In nursing homes, the supply of vitamins is therefore often disastrous. 80% are not even getting the minimum supply required by the RDA. Older people are thus susceptible to infections. The following nutrients are most needed by the elderly. If your parents live in a retirement home, you should give them a nutrient supplement subscription for Christmas.

10 million diabetics need more micronutrients

In 2010 there will be 10 million diabetics in Germany. They will cost the health insurance system 37 billion euros annually. Every third person will become diabetic when they reach old age. It is the third leading cause of death in the Western world. The non-hereditary type 2 diabetes is in 95% of cases self-inflicted. Obesity is the main cause of diabetes. Lowering the weight in the early stages of diabetis will immediately control the sugar and will thus result in a drop in blood pressure and blood fats. Therefore, the best way to prevent diabetes is to stay slim or lose weight. This is the simple and cruel truth in a country where every second person is overweight.

Prevention through micronutrients?
Vitamin D greatly reduces the risk of diabetes by 33%, as shown in studies

---

FACTS

A micronutrient program for the elderly

Information on daily intake:
- 400-800 IU vitamin D for bone protection and to lower the risk of cancer.
- 1000 µg of vitamin B$_{12}$ for mental performance, immune system and formation of blood cells.
- A multivitamin supplement that contains 400 µg folic acid against anemia and for the protection of blood vessels and brain.
- 100 µg of vitamin E against cardiovascular disease.
- 1000 mg vitamin C for the immune system, to protect the eyes, brain and blood vessels.
- 1000 mg calcium for the bones.
- 350 mg of magnesium. Not to be taken together with calcium! Magnesium is best taken in the evening; it makes for a good night's sleep.
- 70-100 mcg selenium as a protection against cancer.
- 5 times per day fruits and vegetables.
- 100% pure vegetable juices or fresh out of the bottle for additional antioxidant phytochemicals. Please select the lowest possible salt content (sodium) in finished products. Salt tends to increase blood pressure.

with 83,779 women.[163] Is it really surprising that a deficiency of vitamin D results in an increased risk for diabetes?

In 4 trials with 147,000 participants more magnesium decreased the risk of diabetes by about 30%.[164, 165, 166, 167] All this is convincing, but it distracts from the actual problem: more and more people are eating themselves to death! Every third euro spent in the health care system is a result of obesity.

Vascular damage - the main problem

Antioxidants can at least help to alleviate the consequent damages of diabetes. The problem with diabetes: due to a strong insulin resistance sugar in the blood stream is no longer packed into the cells. The "unpacked" residual sugar, which under the influence of free radicals combines with proteins (glycation), then attacks your transport system - the large and small blood vessels. An additional, concomitant high blood pressure, which three-quarters of all people with diabetes have, now damages these vessels by additional pressure. This damage affects the finest capillaries of the eyes, kidneys, feet, nerves and heart. The sad consequence of diabetes-induced vascular damage in Germany per year: 6,000 cases of blindness, 20,000 patients on dialysis for kidney failure, 27,000 amputations, intolerable nerve pain (diabetic neuropathy), 44,000 strokes and 27,000 heart attacks.

Reducing vascular damage through antioxidants

Sugar molecules circulating in the blood react with proteins and then thicken the vascular walls by inclusions leading to damage in various organs. Vitamin C can reduce this sugar-protein reaction by 33%.[168, 169] Thus the vascular damage decreases. In addition, vitamin C protects your eyes, which are particularly vulnerable to damaged blood vessels. Diabetics produce significantly more free radicals than other people and thus get more ofter free radical diseases. The risk of cardiovascular disease for example is five times higher. In smokers with diabetes this increases the risk even 20-fold! This is due to the extra free radicals from cigarette smoke.

Test the destruction caused by free radicals

Many diabetics do not believe that they are particularly affected by free radicals and have an increased need for antioxidants. The most convincing proof is then the measurement of cell damage caused by free radical by means of an MDA test (see page 25).

GOOD TO KNOW
Micronutrient blood levels
Low blood levels commonly indicate a low micronutrient content in the cells. You can tune your blood micronutrient levels in the upper third of the norm in order to achieve optimal performance and immune function. With this your tissue storage will fill up gradually.

The higher the number of perforated cell membranes due to free radicals bombardment, the clearer it is that you have an increased need for antioxidants.

The immune system of diabetics

Why do diabetics excrete micronutrients?

In the case of gradually failing kidneys of diabetics, many micronutrients are excreted too rapidly or are not retained. This leads to symptoms of deficiency that put a burden on the immune system. The following placebo-controlled study is interesting: one group received a multivitamin-/multimineral preparation, the other a placebo. In the diabetic patients who took the vitamin-mineral supplement, the risk of infection decreased by 82% within one year.[170]

Sport and micronutrients

Why are free radicals created during aerobic sports?

Endurance sports lead to a 30-fold increase in oxygen consumption. Everywhere where oxygen is consumed or transported, free radicals are created. If they are not sufficiently bound by antioxidant vitamins there is a risk of damage to muscle cells and cell membranes. This transient structural damage to cell membranes and DNA can be shown in different test procedures.[171] The damage is usually repaired by the body within days.

Since antioxidant vitamins can significantly reduce the damage caused by free radicals[172], the recovery phase after exercise is significantly reduced.

On a diet: Vitamin deficiency is bound to occur

Why do you receive fewer micronutrients when you are on a diet?

Many, especially younger women, suffer from a vitamin deficiency because of their diet crazes. Due to the reduced intake of calories, the supply of micronutrients is of course also reduced. This micronutrient deficiency weakens the immune system, reduces your performance and leads to emotional instability and depression due to lack of micronutrients for the nerves.

Women who diet suffer more frequently from pain and mood swings before menstruation (premenstrual syndrome, PMS). In studies this could be improved significantly with magnesium and vitamin B_6. I have already described the folate deficiency in 99% of women of childbearing age and its terrible consequences (page 99). The effects are dramatically exacerbated once dieting starts. When

> **GOOD TO KNOW**
>
> **Test your personal needs**
> The governmental intake recommendations do not take into consideration biochemical individuality and genetic differences. With various blood tests you can get clarity! If an MDA blood test for example, shows that you have compromised cell membranes (antioxidant deficiency), or that your homocysteine levels are too high (B-vitamin deficiency), or that you are in the lower third of the normal value for other micronutrients, you should act, even if you perhaps meet the minimum intake recommendations.

an unplanned pregnancy occurs during dieting such a deficiency can no longer be compensated in the short term and may lead to malformations of the child.

Genetic factors – your biochemical individuality

What does genetic material have to do with vitamin requirements?

Depending on your genetic makeup, the micronutrient needs vary enormously. This is also known as "biochemical individuality", because the metabolism of various people is significantly different. Two examples:

as early as in 1967, animal studies demonstrated precisely that the necessary vitamin C requirement to prevent scurvy can fluctuate 8-fold[173]. In humans, this means: for purely genetic reasons, the vitamin C requirement –

depending on the individual metabolism – can be 75-400 mg daily.
Certain genetic defects can result in a significantly increased requirement
of certain micronutrients. For example, 18% of the French population has
a certain genetic variation (HLA-B35-deficiency)[174], which leads to less
magnesium being stored in the cells. However magnesium plays a crucial role
in hundreds of metabolic processes.

People with high blood fat levels

Many healthy people already have high blood fat levels at a young age.
Although high blood fats represent a long-term risk factor, not many people
wish to reduce it with medication. Then at least you should lower the blood
fat with vitamin B_3 (nicotinic acid).

A study of vitamin B_3 with 8,341 patients showed that this vitamin is
the only substance that lowers triglycerides by 52% and cholesterol by 22%.
Even the lipoprotein A, another independent factor in the pathogenesis
of cardiovascular disease, could be decreased with this.[175] The long-term
evaluation of the study after 15 years resulted in a decrease of 11% in mortality
when using vitamin B_3 compared with other lipid-lowering treatments.[176]

The National Institute of Health (NIH) in the U.S. named vitamin B_3
as one of three effective methods in the national "Cholesterol Lowering
Program" to lower blood fats.[177]

An analysis, which studies on cholesterol - lowering medications are
most frequently cited, is very interesting: cholesterol-lowering agents, which
are provided with a patent, are mentioned 8x more frequently than the
unpatentable vitamin B_3.[178] Patents mean more money for pharmaceutical
companies. The pharmaceutical industry therefore never fails to tell all doctors
and journalists time and again that Vitamin B_3 is not well tolerated and that
it causes temporary redness of the skin or flushes after one takes it. If you
ever ask your doctor about vitamin B_3, he will most likely recite that first. Of
course that's completely outdated. If you combine vitamin B_3 with Inositol,
another B vitamin, it never leads to skin flushes. Vitamin B_3 will then be more
compatible than any other blood lipid lowering agents on the market. Since
pharmaceutical companies no longer deny the positive effect of vitamin B_3,
products came onto the market that combine statins – a lipid lowering agent
- with vitamin B_3. It has been proven in many studies that these combination
products work much better on blood lipids than statins alone.[179,180] Whether
this works better than vitamin B_3 alone was not examined in studies, but –
looking at the logic - in the combination the product at least is patentable.

Medicines influence the absorption of micronutrients

Some medications use the existing micronutrients in the body to be broken down and metabolized. They can also block or flush micronutrients. Aspirin for example decreases the exretion of vitamin C from the body 10-fold and interferes with the vitamin C transport. Gastric acid buffers and certain antibiotics block most of the water-soluble B-vitamins.

Medicines alter the secretion or transport of micronutrients. This is an extremely abbreviated list to serve just as a brief demonstration of how medicines can influence the absorption of micronutrients.

Drug / Stimulants	Vitamin / Mineral
Alcohol, antibiotics, gastric acid buffers	B_2
Alcohol, gastric acid buffers, corticosteroids, Penicillin	B_6
Alcohol, nicotine, birth control pill, drugs for malaria prophylaxis, antibiotics, gastric acid buffers, barbiturates	Folate
Antibiotics (by the destruction of the intestinal flora that builds B12), stomach buffers, antihistamines, anti-diabetics, aspirin, birth control pill	B_{12}
Nicotine, high caffeine, aspirin, antibiotics, birth control pill	C
Gastric acid buffer, aspirin	A
Antibiotics, alcohol, tetracycline, diuretic, Neuroleptics	Magnesium

Special case: Chemotherapy

Do you need more micronutrients during chemotherapy?

Many patients are very interested in their nutrition and vitamins when they have cancer. Often the patients are told that they should refrain from taking any additional vitamins and antioxidants during chemotherapy. The reason most often given is that the chemotherapy should not be affected by the intake of antioxidants. The latest survey analysis of 19 clinical studies[181] however concluded that none of the studies showed a reduction of the effect of chemotherapy. In fact, some studies showed longer survival times, fewer side effects and improved chemotherapy effect. The reason: because chemotherapy drugs interfere with the transport of vitamins in the body this leads to many unnecessary side effects that are quite similar to the classic symptoms of vitamin deficiency: tiredness, lethargy, headaches, mood swings...

Besides, chemotherapy also causes very unpleasant side effects, as in the case of neuropathy – painful damage to the nervous system – which can be reduced by the intake of B-vitamins.

Selenium enhances the effect of chemotherapeutic agents

Prof. Beuth heads the "Institute for Scientific Evaluation of naturopathic methods" in Cologne, Germany. His academic field is the evaluation of complementary cancer therapies that are used concomitantly with chemo- and radiotherapy. In an interview I did recently with Prof. Beuth on selenium, he states: "until recently, the use of antioxidants was always disputed by oncologists and radiation therapists. They would say, 'careful with selenium and other antioxidants', because the chemo and radiation therapies are based on oxidative effects. If antioxidant substances are administered simultaneously, 'you reduce the effect of chemotherapy and radiotherapy'. We now know very well that this is not the case – even at the molecular level. That means that we can now safely say that selenium does not block the chemo-and radiotherapy treatment, quite the contrary, their effectiveness improved."

Amalgam – micronutrients help to detoxify

Amalgam is in everyone's mouths. 90 million amalgam dental fillings are placed each year in Germany. Amalgam dental fillings are highly contaminated with mercury, a toxic heavy metal. A study by the University of Tübingen shows that 30% of all Germans have a higher mercury concentration in their saliva than what is allowed by the limits of the World Health Organization (WHO). In Sweden, amalgam dental fillings have already been banned.

A person with amalgam fillings takes in about eight to 10 mg of mercury per day. The mercury is deposited in the kidneys and the brain and accumulates in the gums. The mercury concentration increases with the size of the filling, the number of fillings, the age of the fillings and the age of those affected. It takes about 18 years for mercury to be discarded from the body. The older the fillings are, the more mercury is released.

A chewing-gum test can determine how much mercury from your amalgam-landfill escapes in the mouth. Many laboratories offer this mercury gum test.

The effects of mercury

The immune system:

Selenium binds itself to heavy metals and neutralizes these. Thus selenium reserves are used up because of mercury detoxification. Therefore, people with amalgam fillings have an increased selenium requirement. When there is a selenium deficiency, heavy metals cannot be transported from the body. In addition, the immune system suffers greatly from a selenium deficiency. With mercury exposure the number of natural killer cells often decreases and the strength of the B-and T-lymphocytes may be reduced.[182]

Fertility:
Mercury accumulates in the placenta. Women with high mercury levels often suffer from hormone disorders.[183] Mercury competes with zinc in the body. For example, there where zinc should be incorporated into enzymes, it is blocked by mercury. Zinc is also important for the synthesis of various hormones and in men for example for the maturation and motility of the sperm.[184] Low zinc levels in the blood are directly linked to low sperm counts and low testosterone levels. Various studies show that an additional intake of zinc can lead to an increased sperm count, improved testosterone production and twice the pregnancy rate in long-standing infertility.[185] Currently 15% of young couples have an unfulfilled desire for children. The zinc deficiency caused by mercury is often to blame for this.

Neurodegenerative diseases:
People who suffer from Alzheimer's disease, multiple sclerosis and Parkinson's disease, often have too low selenium levels and to high mercury levels in the brain. In case of a selenium-deficiency, mercury accumulates in the brain.[186, 187, 188]

Increased need for micronutrients due to amalgam
If you have amalgam fillings, you need more micronutrients because mercury produces free radicals. This creates an increased need for vitamin C, vitamin E and potent antioxidants from fruits and vegetables. There are also significantly higher zinc and selenium requirements.

Amalgam-Removal
During amalgam removal, a lot of mercury enters the body and is deposited there for 15 to 20 years. This is the reason for the increased cancer rate among dentists who over the years have inhaled mercury vapors. Under no circumstances should you seek to remove amalgam fillings during pregnancy!

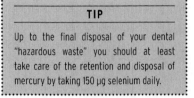

TIP

Up to the final disposal of your dental "hazardous waste" you should at least take care of the retention and disposal of mercury by taking 150 µg selenium daily.

The mercury contamination can be reduced by selenium and DMPS, a substance that binds mercury. In this way mercury can be eliminated via the kidneys and thus does not accumulate in the body.

Only let an expert remove your fillings by simultaneously using heavy metal binding trace elements. For the elimination of heavy metals in the reconstruction and disposal of the fillings, it is advisable to take 400 µg of selenium, 40 mg zinc and 1500 mg of vitamin C daily for one week before and up to two weeks after the dental appointment. Vitamin C activates the excretion of mercury. Ask your pharmacist for specific products. Two weeks after the removal, you should reduce the dosage of trace elements again: do not take more than 200 µg of selenium and no more than 15 mg of zinc per day for extended periods. Trace elements have a narrow upper limit.

Pollution that stresses your body

In the 20th century, the exposure to environmental toxins has increased so dramatically that we can barely control the consequences of exposure any more. This is reflected in the growing toxic sediments in water, soil, air, in food, animals and plants. Pollutants do not stop at the home or office door. Depending on life and work, we lead a life amongst the emissions of chemical molecules from varnishes, carpets, selants, fillers, adhesives, high-tech building materials, computers & copiers, fumes from the smoke of cigarettes among others. Micronutrients can to a small degree bind different pollutants and promote their excretion.

Pollution in the environment

In the past 20 years, the number of chemical compounds in the environment has increased from 2 to 7 million! The pollution of soil, water and air is on the rise. This also increases the storage of pollutants in the brain and adipose tissue, in which chemical compounds can be deposited for up to 20 years. Particularly heavy metals burden our system because they bind to specific proteins and enzymes and thereby affect their function. The heavy metals are stored in various organs and accumulate there. Our daily uptake is e.g. 200 to 300 µg of lead and 25 to 30 µg of cadmium. Even the small increase of 10 µg/dl of lead in children's blood causes a decrease of up to 5 points in an IQ Test.[189] The values of mercury in the brains of Alzheimer's and Parkinson's patients are significantly elevated.

Also through seemingly innocuous food packaging such as beverage and food cans metals accumulate in our body that do not belong there. Aluminum for example is stored in the brain and is a factor in the development of Alzheimer's disease.

Pollution around the house

When speaking of environmental stress, most people think of industrial plants and automobile emissions. But we spend 80% of our time indoors. A few examples of pollution in the office:

- Computer: brominated dibenzofuranes as flame retardants.
- Printer: benzene, styrene, nitroarenes, nitropyrene, trinitro fluro.
- Copier: toner particulates, ozone.
- Paint and felt pens, glue: solvents, aromatic compounds, styrene, xylenes, toluene, ethyl acetate.
- Monitors: a permanent magnetic and high ionizing radiation exposure.
- Carpet: vaporizing insecticides (pyrethroids) and fungal agents.
- Wood: fungicides, insecticides, solvents.
- Furniture and Leather: formaldehyde and carboxyl groups.
- Thermal insulation products: polychlorinated biphenyls, formaldehyde.
- Cleaning agents: tensides, phosphates, formaldehyde, p-dichlorobenzene, etc.
- Textiles: pesticides, dyes, tetrachloroethene and heavy metals which are absorbed through the skin.
- Cigarette smoking is the strongest room air pollutant

In the U.S. the symptoms caused by the pollution in rooms are called "sick building syndrome". Performance drops by 10-20% because of this.

People who work in factories or with chemical cleaners, and most craft occupations are exposed to an even higher burden, often develop a "multi-chemical sensitivity".

Evidence of pollution

The "sick building syndrome" and "multi-chemical sensitivity" are not psychosomatic diseases, but can be measured in the laboratory. Hair mineral analysis and special blood tests can determine how much pollution you have already picked up. The increase of oxidative damage to cell membranes and to the genetic material (see page 25) can be measured.[190] Analyses of the air in the rooms, house dust and certain materials may reveal disease-causing pollutants at home.

INFO

High pollutant concentrations can be found especially at home or in the office. 50,000 chemicals and 3,000 preservatives are used around the house.

Pollutants in allergy and asthma sufferers

Many diseases such as allergies, asthma and skin diseases are closely linked to pollution. 9% of school children in large cities suffer from asthma, 20% from dermatitis and 15% from hay fever. The number of adults with asthma has doubled in the past 20 years. There are 8 million people in Germany who suffer from asthma. 18.7 million or 8.2% of the population suffer from asthma in the U.S.

A co-factor for asthma is the reaction of an overactive immune system.[193] The body's own immune messenger substance histamine is responsible for the allergic symptoms. To fight these symptoms, medicine – anti-histamines – can be taken. But these make you tired.

> **GOOD TO KNOW**
>
> **Vitamin C for allergies and asthma**
> Asthma and allergy sufferers often have low blood levels of vitamin C[191], which is involved in histamine degradation. Studies show that 2,000-5,000 mg vitamin C per day could reduce histamine by 38%. Seven studies show a reduction of asthma attacks through vitamin C.[192] In addition, calcium reduces the release of histamine. The combination of calcium + vitamin C can prevent sun allergies, which 15% of women suffer from. But you should already start filling the calcium deposits 1-2 weeks before the holiday in the sun.

Binding of pollutants through minerals and trace elements

Undesirable heavy metals are particularly easily absorbed in to the body when blood levels of essential minerals and trace elements are low. Accordingly, heavy metal absorption can be reduced if sufficient quantities of calcium, copper, iron, zinc and selenium are present. When there is a sufficient supply of zinc, cadmium is excreted from the body. Calcium binds lead, so it can be eliminated. Selenium disposes of mercury, aluminum, cadmium and lead.[194]

Heavy metals and chemical compounds produce a flood of free radicals in the body that deplete antioxidants. The many chemical compounds that must be disposed of by the body therefore result in a measurable decrease in the antioxidant vitamins. The levels of zinc and selenium, which are needed for the production of endogenous antioxidant enzymes, also decrease.

Binding of pollutants by vitamin C

Nitrate compounds enter our food chain through drinking water because of fertilizers. However, water filters can remove nitrates. Even food additives such as E 250 to E 252 (sodium nitrite) and cigarette smoke contribute to nitrate

> **TIP**
>
> You can hardly escape pollutants. Detoxify: minerals and trace elements support the disposal of pollutants. Antioxidants at least reduce the burden of free radicals.

pollution Smokers often have four times the normal amounts of nitrate in their blood. 90% of the nitrosamines that are transformed from nitrate compounds in the body are triggers for cancer.

Vitamin C prevents the conversion of nitrates into cancer-causing nitrosamines. This could explain the protective effect of vitamin C against cancer at high pollution levels. To effectively dispose of the 60 to 150 mg daily nitrate intake means that a considerable part of the vitamin C is depleted.

Vitamin C also promotes the excretion of mercury and lead. Thus, through the use of vitamin C, the lead levels of smokers can be reduced by 80%.[195] A study of 4,213 adolescents found that the adolescents with the highest vitamin C blood levels had 89% less elevated lead blood levels.[196] To dispose of nitrates and heavy metals it seems beneficial to take more vitamin C.

Conclusion: 80% of the population belongs to several risk groups.

If you do not smoke, drink, do not exercise, are not pregnant, neither take the pill nor are on a diet, if you are not over 65 (with mal-absorption) or younger than 15 years old (growth phase), if you do not have any chronic diseases, are not suffering from bowel problems, never take medicines, eat ecologically wholesome food directly from the field, if you never eat in cafeterias or when you are on a business trip, if you live in a pollution free environment, clean your house only with vinegar and never work on computers, if you live in a stress-free meditative calm state, then the low recommended daily allowance values (RDA) are no problem for you. I congratulate you! You must live on an idyllic island in the Pacific. Thus, your highly-sensitive cells and organs are protected against pollutants and free radicals, and enzymatic repair processes can be executed. Everyone else may need more than the minimum levels of the RDA.

GOOD TO KNOW

Safe intake rather than minimal intake

Three quarters of the population have a higher need but are categorized in the "small print" of the RDA. Recent genetic studies also show that the vitamin requirements vary greatly between different individuals. A down-to-the milligram calculated intake recommendation is therefore absurd. The "safe intake" is approximately 3 to 5 times higher than the minimum intake recommendation of the RDA. An optimal micronutrient intake helps your health several times over:

· It ensures that all metabolic processes work optimally.
· It ensures that the immune system is strong.
· It ensures that tissue stores are well filled.

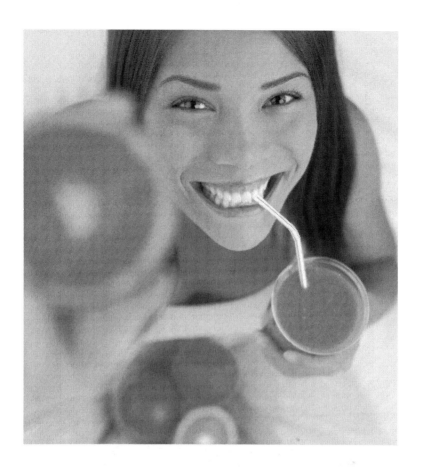

CHAPTER 6

Your personal micronutrient program

Can you overdose on vitamins? How safe are vitamins? Why can trace elements be overdosed? Why is it not allowed to make claims regarding health in the package insert?

Product qualitity

I advise you to stay away from no-name products or products by unknown companies from the internet. Often the ingredients are declared incorrectly and there are no certificates. The bioavailability of the products is often poor, because the chemical formulation is inferior. Market leaders are usually under strict observation by their competitors thus they are often a better choice.

Quality products also use more expensive raw materials, for example mixed carotenes from natural spirulina algae, which contain five different carotenes rather than cheap synthetic beta-carotene, or natural vitamin E, which is more effective than artificial vitamin E. These quality raw materials differ significantly from cheap products in the production price.

Multi-vitamins & minerals or single supplements?

Vitamins, minerals and trace elements work together and are interdependent. The result can only be as strong as the weakest link in the chain. Therefore, it is best to take them in a combination of micronutrients – as a micronutrient complex. This ensures that there really are no gaps.

Only with the antioxidants vitamin C and vitamin E (for additional cell protection), selenium (as selenium is rarely included in Multivitamin-/Mineral pills) it makes sense to buy additional micronutrient products.

Information gaps in package inserts

Have you actually ever read on your vitamin D from the supermarket, a statement like this: "vitamin D lowers risk of heart attacks by 40%"? No? Quite simply, it is forbidden to make medical claims concerning vitamin supplements. For the same reason your probiotic yoghurt does not contain the statement "strengthens the immune system in the intestine". This medical statement would make the the yogurt a pharmacy-only product.

To be able to use medical statements, you need an expensive drug approval. Since vitamins are no longer patentable, this investment is not interesting for any vitamin manufacturer. Thus you will not find any documentation or packaging inserts that would alert you as a consumer that vitamins prevent certain diseases or can be used therapeutically.

How do you dose properly?

Consumers are of course most interested in the practical aspects concerning vitamin use. But especially the tabloid press often irritates consumers with stories about over-dosing. But what are the facts?

Fat- and water-soluble vitamins

Vitamins are divided into two major groups: the fat- and water-soluble. The first group includes, for example, vitamins A and D, the second group includes B-vitamins and vitamin C.

Why can you overdose on fat-soluble vitamins? And why is it difficult to overdose on water-soluble vitamins?

Fat-soluble vitamins can be stored in fat and accumulate there. That makes a vitamin A and D overdose possible. In contrast, an excess of water-soluble vitamins is simply excreted. That's why you can hardly overdose on these. Let me give you some examples:

- Even the German nutritional society (DGE) confirms: one can easily take up to 10,000 mg vitamin C per day. However, the disproportionately low-DGE recommendation is 100 mg.
- With Vitamin B_1: 10,000 times the amount of the RDA can be taken without major side effects.[197]
- An overdose of vitamin D is possible only in theory because fat-soluble vitamins are stored. In fact, the vitamin D deficiency is so great that milk is enriched with vitamin D in many countries. 90% of Germans suffer from vitamin D deficiency. Older people almost always have a vitamin D deficiency.
- Vitamin A can also be overdosed, because it is fat-soluble. Since beta-carotene is converted into vitamin A in the body, most multi-vitamins contain only a low dosage or no vitamin A but beta-carotene instead.

> **GOOD TO KNOW**
>
> **Optimal vitamin intake**
> The optimal intake is about 3 to 5 times the RDA for water soluble vitamins (C and B-vitamins) for people that do not have chronic diseases or environmental stress. The optimal intake for antioxidants is likely to be 5 to 8-fold the RDA minimum. Especially when it comes to vitamin C, 400 mg is advised by many experts. However, when it comes to minerals and trace elements however one should stick to the RDA and not exceed this considerably. In people with particular stress, chronic disease, acute infection or undergoing chemotherapy more may be needed.

Minerals and trace elements - narrow limits

The safe area for minerals and trace elements is much narrower than that of vitamins. Trace elements have a fine balance in the body.

To get all the essential trace elements, it makes the most sense to switch to whole foods. In the outer layers of grain or nuts the trace elements are optimally combined.

Exceptions are the trace elements zinc, selenium and iodine, which should be added, because the soils in many Northern European countries are poor in those elements. Calcium should also be supplemented, because there is a great deficiency.

Upper and lower limits for a safe intake

In what dose can you take vitamins in the long term?

Column 1 + 2 of the table: for the standardization of policies in the EU, Dr. Derek Shrimpton has, over a period of five years, evaluated over 300 studies[198] to ensure the safety of micronutrient supplements for the consumer. From this data a conservative upper-limit safe intake was formulated. This range is definitely safe for the consumer who adds vitamins and minerals daily in addition to a balanced diet.

Many US consumers supplement higher. The values of Prof. Shrimpton are conservative and for several micronutrients well below the upper limit (U.L.) of the US Food and Nutrition Board which include the total intake of food and supplements together. So in the US you may see these US U.L. more often. These upper limits are unpractical because you would need to deduct your intake from food to get a safe intake from supplements. However the higher US upper limits (folic acid 1000 µg, vitamin E 1000 mg, vitamin D 50 µg) show that supplementation is considered safe.

Also the EFSA (European Food Safety Authority) - Europe's highest authority on food safety - has for six years reviewed all available studies of vitamin safety and has defined maximum limits - the "tolerable upper intake level". Interestingly, they came to similar conclusions. For many B-vitamins there is no upper limit, since they are excreted if they are not used up, and the upper limit for vitamin D is much higher, at 50 µg.

What is the safe maximum intake?

Safe upper-limit for the daily, additional, long-term intake of vitamin- and mineral supplements according to Prof. Shrimpton		German RDA* (minimum intake)	How many times the RDA is still safe
Fat-soluble vitamins			
A	2,300 µg	1,000 µg	2.3-times
D	20 µg or 800 IE	5 µg or 200 IE	4-times
Vitamins with additional antioxidative function			
Beta-Carotene	20 mg	2 mg	10-times
E	400 mg	14 mg	28-times
C	2,000 mg	100 mg	27-times
Water-soluble vitamins			
B$_1$ (Thiamine)	100 mg	1.2 mg	83-times
B$_2$ (Riboflavin)	200 mg	1.4 mg	142-times
B$_3$ (Niacin)	450 mg	16 mg	28-times
B$_5$ (Pantothenic acid)	500 mg	6 mg	84-times
B$_6$ (Pyridoxine)	200 mg	1.5 mg	133-times
B$_7$ (Biotin)	500 mg	-	
Folate / Folic acid	800 µg	400 µg	2-times
B$_{12}$ (Cobalamine)	500 µg	3 µg	166-times
Minerals / Trace elements			
Calcium	1,500 mg	1,000 mg	1.5-times
Magnesium	350 mg	350 mg	-
Iron	15 mg	10 mg	1.5-times
Iodine	500 µg	200 µg	2.5-times
Zinc	15 mg	10 mg	1.5-times
Phosphor	1,500 mg	700 mg	2.1-times
Copper	5 mg	1-1.5 mg	3-times
Chrome	200 µg	30-100 µg	2-times
Manganese	15 mg	2-5 mg	3-times
Selenium	200 µg	30-70 µg	2.8-times
Molybdenum	200 µg	50-100 µg	2-times

* German RDA (DGE) - recommendation: example for men between 25 and 51 years of age.

135

Column 3: since the German RDA values include neither an increased need nor preventive aspects, they do not correspond with the optimal intake. Therefore I have only outlined the German RDA-values in the table (the recommendations

> **TIP**
>
> In fat-soluble vitamins, trace elements and minerals you need to watch and calculate if you combine several products so you do not exceed the upper limits.

for men 21-55 years of age) for comparison. The RDA represents the minimum that should not be fallen short of for a longer period of time. Again: the minimum is not the optimum.

Column 4: indicates by how much you can exceed the German RDA value in the long-term with micronutrient supplements. For vitamin B_{12} for example the continued safe upper-limit intake amount is 166 times (!) the German RDA recommendation. In the long run this means that you can take these vitamins for many years. You would have to devour vitamin pills, on a daily and permanent basis to reach this upper limit for most B-vitamins.

Although 125 million Americans are currently taking vitamins, in eight years the National Poison Control Center has reported very few serious cases of vitamin overdose. Even in five years of liberal legislation in the UK no cases of overdose are known.

The safe framework for your individual intake

Your metabolism and your immune system do not take breaks. You need to continuously and daily replenish it with essential biomaterials. Some examples: when you catch a virus a vitamin C deficiency results in an unnecessary cold. With a vitamin B deficiency, you may have mood swings, stage a superfluous "relationship drama" and live with a high risk of cardiovascular disease. Once you have used up all water-soluble vitamins, a small part can temporarily be stored and the remainder is excreted without a problem. The values of the table form a framework within which you can move around without worry. A safe intake that will always provide your body with adequate levels of micronutrients. With the results of clinical trials for cardiovascular disease, cancer, osteoporosis, dementia, cataracts, I've tried to give you clues as to which intake provides long-term protection.

The nonsense of "milligram-specific" recommendations

Most readers would now like to know what intake of additional vitamins, minerals and trace elements would be appropriate. My answer:

all the factors that determine your life also set your vitamin and mineral requirements. Let's take a look at the course of any week: maybe you work in an office and have polluted amalgam fillings.

> **TIP**
>
> The concept of a milligram-specific, standardized allowance for everyone does not correspond with reality. Your individual need is crucial. What your micronutrient need is, actually depends on several factors: personal lifestyle, age, existing illnesses, additional burdens, individual metabolism, genetic factors, nutrition and environmental pollution.

On Monday you smoke twice as much as usual and thereby use up most antioxidants. On Tuesday your immune system fights and defeats a virus with an enormous vitamin C consumption. On Wednesday and Thursday you eat micronutrient-poor food downtown, on Friday, due to chronic stress, you have an increased vitamin B requirement; on Saturday afternoon, you do aerobics and sweat out lots of minerals. In the evening you drink a lot of alcohol and deplete most vitamin B1; at night you have an increased loss of zinc because you had sex with your wife, and on Sunday you take aspirin, which leads to a 10-fold washout of vitamin C. So what is the right intake for this person?

To get to the milligram-exact intake recommendation, a genetic average citizen is constructed with a standardized way of life, in order to set some intake value. This concept is completely absurd. It makes more sense to set a framework for a "safe intake" which covers your needs in all situations. You know your personal situation best.

The problem with micronutrients today is not that a large portion of the population takes too many vitamins, but the serious health consequences of micronutrient deficiencies due to poor nutrition.

An optimal supply of micronutrients can make a big difference. In the short term: how you feel, how well your metabolism works and how effectively you can fight infection. Remember: you can only feel as good as your metabolism works. Put junk food in and you will only get minimal performance out of your wonderfull biochemical engine – your body. In my experience the short term benefits can really motivate many people because you just feel better and get fewer infections. In the long term an adaquate micronutrient intake and good nutrition protects you and your health from various diseases. There is no better insurance policy for your health.

References

1   Murray, M.: Encyclopedia of Nutritional Supplements. Prima Publishing 1996; 7–8.
2   Wie ticken die Ärzte. Spiegel. 2007; Jan: 132–33.
3   Pryor, W.A., et al.: Vitamin E and heart disease: basic science to clinical intervention trials. Free Radic Biol. Med. 2000; 28: 141–164.
4   Stampfer, M., et al.: Vitamin E consumption and the risk of coronary heart disease in women. New England J. Med. 1993; 328: 1444–1449.
5   Grey, K., et al.: Inverse correlation be-tween plasma vitamin E and mortality from ischemic heart disease in cross cultural epidemiology. Am. J. Clin. -Nutr. 1991; 53: 326S-334S.
6   Stampfer, M., et al.: Vitamin E consumption and the risk of coronary heart disease in women. New England J. Med., 1993; 328: 1444–1449.
7   Rimm, E., et al.: Vitamin E consump-tion and the risk of coronary heart dis-ease in men. New England J. Med. 1993; 328: 1450–1456.
8   Mehta J.: Intake of antioxidants among american cardiologists. Am J Cardiol 1997; 79: 1558–1560.
9   Stephens, et al.: Randomized controlled trial of vitamin E in patients with coronary heart disease. Lancet 1996; 347: 781–786.
10 Ridker, P., Stampfer, M., et al.: Inflammation, aspirin and the risk of cardiovascular disease in apparently healthy men. N. Engl. J. Med. 1997; 336: 975–979.
11 Rimm E., et al.: Vitamin E consumption and the risk of coronary heart disease in men. N. Engl. J. Med. 1993 (328), 1450–1456
12 Stampfer M., et al.: Vitamin E consumption and the risk of coronary heart disease in women. N. Eng. J. Med. 1993; 328, 1444–1449.
13 Knekt, P., et al.: Am. J. Epid.1994; 139: 1180
14 Losonczy, K., Harris, T.B., et al.: Vitamin E and vitamin C supplement use and the risk of all cause coronary heart disease mortality in older persons. Am. J. Clin. Nutr. 1996, 64: 190–196.
15 Hu, F., Stampfer, M.J., et al.: Dietary intake of alpha-linolenic acid and risk of fatal ischemic heart disease among women. Am. J. Clin. Nutr. 1999; 69: 890–7.
16 Hu, F., Stampfer, M.J., et al.: Dietary intake of alpha-linolenic acid and risk of fatal ischemic heart disease among women. Am. J. Clin. Nutr. 1999; 69: 890–7.
17 Brigelius-Flohe, Leist, Gassmann, Schultz, et al.: Novel Urinary Metabolite of Alpha-Tocopherol, 2,5,7,8,-Tetra-methyl-2 (2'-Carboxyethyl)-6-Hydroxychroman, as an Indicator of Adequate Vitamin E Supply. Am. J. Clin. Nutr. 1995; 62 -(Suppl): 1527S–1534S.
18 Rimm, E., Osganian, S.K., et al.: Vitamin C and risk of coronary heart disease in women. J. Am. Col. Cardiol. 2003; 42: 253–5.
19 Enstrom, J., et al.: Vitamin C intake and mortalily among a sample of the United States population. Epidemiology 1992; 3: 194–202.
20 Knekt P. et al.: Antioxidant vitamins and coronary heart disease risk: a pooled analysis if 9 cohorts. Am. J. Clin. Nutr. 2004; 80: 1508–20.
21 Yokoyama, T.: Serum vitamin C concentration was inversely associated with subsequent 20-year incidence of stroke in a Japanese rural community. The Shibata study. Stroke. 2000; 31(10): 2287–2294.
22 Boekholdt, S., et al.: Plasma concentrations of ascorbic acid and C-reactive protein and the risk of future coronary artery disease, in apparently healthy men and women: the Epic Norfolk prospective population study. Br. J. Nutr. 2006; 96: 516–22.
23 Levine, M., et al.: A new recommended dietary allowance of vitamin C for healthy young women. Proc. Nat. Acad. Sci. USA. 2001; 98: 9842–9846.
24 Flores-Mateo, G., et al.: Selenium and coronary heart disease: a meta analysis. Am. J. Clin. Nutr. 2006; 84: 762–73.
25 Homocystein Lowering Trialists Coop-eration. Dose dependent effects of folic acid on blood concentrations of Homocystein: a meta-analysis of the rand-omized trials. Am. J. Clin. Nutr. 2005; 82: 806–12.
26 Stampfer, M., et al.: Vitamin intervention for stroke prevention trial: an efficacy analysis. Stroke. 2005; 36: 2404–9.
27 He, K., et al.: Folate, vitamin B_6, and B_{12} intakes in relation to risk of stroke among men. Stroke. 2004; 35: 169–74.

28   Rimm, E., et al.: Folate and vitamin B_6 from diet and supplements in relation to risk of coronary heart disease among women. JAMA 1998; 279: 359–364.

29   Willett, W., et al.: Folate and vitamin B_6 from diet and supplements in relation to risk of coronary heart disease among women. JAMA. 1998; 279: 359–64.

30   He, K., et al.: Folate, vitamin B_6 , and B_{12} intakes in relation to risk of stroke among men. Stroke. 2004; 35: 169–74.

31   Wang, X., et al.: Efficacy of folic acid supplementation in stroke prevention: a meta-analysis. Lancet. 2007; 369: 1876–82.

32   Voutilainen, S.: Serum homocysteine, folate and risk of stroke: Kuopio Ischaemic Heart Disease Study. Eur J Cariovasc. Prev. 2005; 12: 369–75.

33   Stampfer, M., et al.: Folate intake and the risk of incident of hypertension among US women. JAMA. 2005; 293: 320–9.

34   Spence, J.D., et al.: Vitamin Intervention for stroke prevention trial: an efficacy analysis. Stroke 2005; 36: 2404–9.

35   Ascherio, A., Rimm, E., et al: Fruit and vegetable intake in relation to risk of ischemic stroke. JAMA.1999; 6: 1233–1239.

36   Manson, E., et al.: The effects of fruit and vegetable on the risk of coronary heart disease. Ann. Intern. Med. 2001; 134: 1206–14.

37   He, J., et al.: Increased consumption of fruit and vegetable is related to a reduced risk of coronary heart disease: meta-analysis of cohort studies. J. Hum. Hypertens. 2007; 21: 717–28.

38   He, F., et al.: Fruit and vegetable consumption and stroke: meta-analysis of cohort studies. Lancet. 2006;367:320–6.

39   Ascherio, A., Rimm, E., et al: Fruit and vegetable intake in relation to risk of ischemic stroke. JAMA.1999; 6: 1233–1239.

40   Manson, E., et al.: The effects of fruit and vegetable on the risk of coronary heart disease. Ann. Intern. Med. 2001; 134: 1206–14.

41   U.S.RDA: RDA vs. RDI: Protecting the health of Americans vs. minimizing nutrient needs, RDA 1992; 17.

42   Block, G.: Vitamin C and cancer prevention: The epidemiological evidence. Am. J. Clin. Nutr. 1991; 53: 270S-282S.

43   Garland, C., et al.: Kalzium and vitamin D. Their potential roles in colon and breast cancer prevention. Ann. NY. Acad. Sci. 1999; 889: 107–19.

44   Giovanucci, E., et al.:Prospective study of predictors of vitamin D status and cancer incidence and mortality in men. J. Natl. Cancer Inst. 2006; 98: 451–9.

45   Stampfer, M., et al.: A prospective study of plasma vitamin D metabolites, vitamin D receptor polymorphisms, and prostate cancer. PLOS Med 2007; 4: 103.

46   Skinner, H., et al.: Vitamin D intake and the risk for pancreatic cancer in two cohorts. Cancer Epid. Biomarker Prev. 2006; 15: 1688–95.

47   Gorham, E., et al.: Optimal vitamin D status for colorectal cancer prevention: a quantitative meta analysis. Am. J. Prev. Med. 2007; 210–6.

48   Ahonen, M., et al.: Prostate cancer and prediagnostic serum 25-hydroxyvitamin D levels. Cancer Causes Control. 2000; 11: 847–52.

49   Willett, W., et al.: Intake of dairy product, Kalzium and vitamin D and risk of breast cancer. J. Natl. Cancer Inst. 2002; 94: 1301–11.

50   Larsson, S., et al.: Dietary folate and incidence of ovarian cancer: the Swedish Mammography Cohort. J. Natl. Cancer Inst. 2004; 96: 396–402.

51   Willett, W., et al.: Plasma folate, vitamin B_6, vitamin B_{12}, homocysteine, and risk of breast cancer. J. Natl. Cancer Inst. 2003; 95: 373–80.

52   Willett, W., et al.: Plasma folate, vitamin B_6, vitamin B_{12}, homocysteine, and risk of breast cancer. J. Natl. Cancer Inst. 2003; 95: 373–80.

53   Lajous, M.: Folate, vitamin B_{12} and postmenopausal breast cancer in a prospective study of French women. Cancer Causes Control. 2006; 17: 1209–13.

54   Willett, W., et al.: Intake of dairy product, Kalzium and vitamin D and risk of breast cancer. J. Natl. Cancer Inst. 2002; 94: 1301–11.

55   Kushi, L., et al.: Dietary folate intakem alcohol and risk of breast cancer in a prospective stuy of postmenopausal women. Epidemiology. 2001; 12: 420–8.

56   Dietary folate intake and breast cancer risk: results form the Shanghai Breast Cancer Study. Cancer Res. 2001; 61: 7136–7141.

57 Larsson, S., et al.: Dietary folate and incidence of ovarian cancer: the Swedish Mammography Cohort. J. Natl. Cancer Inst. 2004; 96: 396–402.

58 Stevens, V., et al.: Folate nutrition and prostate cancer incidence in a large cohort of US men. The American Cancer Society Prevention Study. Am. J. Epid. 2006; 163: 986–96.

59 Pelucchi, G., et al.: Dietary folate and risk of prostate cancer in Italy. Cancer Epid. Bio. Prev. 2005; 14: 944–8.

60 Voorrips, L., et al.: A propective cohort study on antioxidants and folate intake and male lung cancer risk. Cancer Epid. Bio. Prev. 2000; 9: 357–65.

61 Willett, W., et al.: The influence of folate and multivitamin use on the familial risk of colon cancer. Cancer Epid. Bio. Prev. 2002; 11: 227–34.

62 Larsson, S., et al.: A prospective study of dietary folate intake and the risk of colorectal cancer: modification by caffeine intake and cigarette smoking. Cancer Epid. Bio. Prev. 2005; 14: 740–3.

63 Terry, P., et al.: Dietary intake of folic acid and colorectal cancer risk in a cohort of women. Int. J. Cancer. 2002; 97: 864–7.

64 Giovanucci, E., et al.: Vitamin B_6 intake, alcohol consumption, and colorectal cancer: a longitudinal population based cohort of women. Gastroenterology. 2005; 128: 1830–1837.

65 Larsson, S., et al.: A prospective study of dietary folate intake and the risk of colorectal cancer: modification by caffeine intake and cigarette smoking. Cancer Epid. Bio. Prev. 2005; 14: 740–3.

66 Allen, M., et al.: Folat intake and colorectal cancer risk: a meta-analytic approach. Int. J. Cancer. 2005; 20: 825–8.

67 Kiremidjian-Schumacher, et al.: Supplementation with selenium and human -immune functions; Effect on cytotoxic lymphocytes and natural killer cells. Biol. Trace Elem. Res. 1994; 41: 115–127.

68 Abraham, M., et al.: Serum selenium and the subsequent risk of prostate cancer. Cancer Epid. Bio. Prev. 2000; 9: 883–7.

69 Zeegers, M., et al.: Toenail selenium lev-els and the subsequent risk of prostate cancer: a propective study. Cancer Epod. Bio. Prev. 2003; 12: 866–71.

70 Willett, W., et al.: Study of prediagnostic selenium level in toenail and the risk of advanced prostate cancer. J. Nat. Cancer. Inst. 1998; 90: 1219–24.

71 Stampfer, M., et al.: A propective study of plasma levels and prostate cancer risk. J. Natl. Cancer Inst. 2004; 96: 696–703.

72 Meyer, F., et al.: Antioxidant vitamin and mineral supplementation and prostate cancer prevention in the SU.VI.MAX trial. Int. J. Cancer. 2005; 116: 182–6.

73 Etminan, M., et al.: Intake of selenium in the prevention of prostate cancer: a systematic review and meta-analysis. Cancer Causes Control. 2005; 16: 1125–31.

74 Ravaglia, G., et al.: Homocysteine and folate as risk factors for dementia and Alzheimer disease. Am. J. Clin. Nutr. 2005; 82: 636–43.

75 Wang, H., et al.: Vitamin B_{12} and -folate in relation to the development of Alzheimer's disease. Neurology. 2001; 56: 1188–94.

76 Ravaglia, G., et al.: Homocysteine and cognitive function in healthy elderly community dwellers in Italy. Am. J. Clin. Nutr. 2003; 77: 668–73.

77 Bryan, J., et al.: Vitamins, cognition and aging: a review. J. Gerontol. B. Psychol. Sci. Soc. 2001; 56: 327–39.

78 Luchsinger, J., et al.: Relation of higher folate intake to lower risk of Alzheimer disease in the elderly. Arch. Neurol. 2007; 64: 86–92.

79 Snowdon, D., et al.: Serum folate and the severity of atrophy of the neocortex in Alzheimer disease: findings from the nun study. Am. J. Clin. Nutr. 2000; 71: 993–8.

80 Engelhart, M., et al.: Dietary intake of antioxidants and risk of Alzheimer disease. JAMA. 2002; 287: 3223–29.

81 Zandi, P., et al.: Reduced risk of Alzheimer disease in users of antioxidant vitamin supplements: the Cache Country Study. Arch. Neurol. 2004; 61: 82–8.

82 Masaki, K., et al.: Association of vitamin E and C supplement use with cognitive function and dementia in elderly men. Neurology. 2000; 28: 54: 1165–72.

83 Maxwell, C., et al.: Supplement use of antioxidants vitamins and subsequent risk of cognitive decline and dementia. Dement Geriatr. Cogn. Disorder. 2005; 20: 45–51.

84 EVS 1998. In: Ernährungsbericht 2000. DGE 2000; 30–50.

85 Shea, B., et al.: Meta-analysis of thera--pies for postmenopausal osteoporosis. Endocr. Rev. 2002; 23: 560–9.

86 Willet, W., et al.: Kalzium intake and the incidence of forearm and hip fractures. Am. J. Nutr. 1999; 127: 1782.1792.

87   Feskanich, D., et al.: Kalzium, vitamin D, milk consumption and hip fracture: a prospective study among menopausal women. Am. J. Clin. Nutr. 2003; 77: 504–11.

88   Shea, B., et al.: Meta-analysis of therapies for postmenopausal osteoporosis. Endocr. Rev. 2002; 23: 560–9.

89   Feskanich, D., et al.: Kalzium, vitamin D, milk consumption and hip fracture: a prospective study among menopausal women. Am. J. Clin. Nutr. 2003; 77: 504–11.

90   Tang, B., et al.: Use of Kalzium in combination with vitamin D supplementation to prevent fractures and bone loss in people aged 50 years and older: a meta-analysis. Lancet. 2007; 370: 657–66.

91   Willett, W., et al.: Fracture prevention with vitamin D supplementation: a meta-analysis of randomized controlled trials. JAMA. 2005; 293: 2257–64.

92   Weber, P.: Vitamin K and bone health. Nutr. 2001; 17: 880–7.

93   Feskanich, D., Willett, C., et al.: Vitamin K and hip fracture in women: a prospective study. Am. J. Clin. Nutr. 1999; 69: 74–9.

94   Tucker, KL., et al.: Dietary Vitamin K intakes are associated with hip fracture but not with bone density in elderly men and women. Am. J. Clin. Nutr. 2000; 71: 1201–8.

95   Adamson, J., et al.: Vitamin K and the prevention of fractures: systematic review and meta-analysis of randomized controlled trials. Arch. Intern. Med. 2006; 166: 1256–61.

96   Adamson, J., et al.: Vitamin K and the prevention of fractures: systematic review and meta-analysis of randomized controlled trials. Arch. Intern. Med. 2006; 166: 1256–61.

97   Ward, K., et al.: A meta-analysis of the effects of cigarette smoking on bone mineral density. Calcif. Tissue. Int. 2001; 68: 259–70.

98   Dietl, H.: Die Bedeutung von Mikronährstoffen. Forum Medizin Verlag, 1999.

99   Seddon, J., et al.: Prospective study of intake of fruits, vegetables, vitamins and carotenoids and risk of age-related mac-ular disease. Arch. Ophthal. 2004; 122: 882–92.

100   Chylack, J.: Epidemiologic Evidence of a Role for the Antioxidanz Vitamins and Carotinoids in Cataract Prevention. Am. J. Clin. Nutr. 1991; 53 (Suppl.): 352S-355S.

101   Swanson, A.: Elemental analysis of normal and cataractous human lens tissue. Biochem. Biophys. Res. Comm. 1971; 45: 1488–1496.

102   Steiner, M.: Das Potential der antioxidativen Vitamine. In: Fortschr. Med. 1994; 112(33): 8.

103   Dietl, H.: Die Bedeutung von Mikronährstoffen. Forum Medizin Verlag, 1999.

104   Thomas, W.R., et al.: Vitamin C and immunity: an assessment of evidence. Clinical Experimental Immunology 1978; 32: 370–379.

105   Bland, J.: Vitamin C – the Future is now. New Canaan: Keats Publishing 1995; 16–17.

106   Chandra, R.: Nutritional regulation of immunity and risk of infection in old age. Immunology. 1989; 67: 141–147.

107   De Weck, A.: Immune response and aging. Constitutive and environmental -aspects. In: Munro, H.: Nutrition of the elderly. New York: Raven Press 1991.

108   Niedermann, M.S.: Respiratory infections in the elderly. New York, Raven Press 1991.

109   Chandra, R.: Effect of vitamin and trace element supplementation on immune -response and infection in elderly subjects. Lancet 1992; 340: 1124–1127.

110   Hofmeister, M.: Auswirkung von alimentären Ergänzungsmitteln auf die Gesundheit. Ernährung und Medizin. 2005; 20: 115–122.

111   Barringer, T., et al.: Effect of a multivitamin and mineral supplement on infection and quality of life. A randomized, double blind, placebo controlled trial. An. Intern. Med. 2003; 138: 365–371.

112   Chandra, R., et al.: Nutrition and Im-mun-ity. Vitamins and Immunomodulation in AIDS. Nutrition 1996; 12: 1–7.

113   Tolmunen, T., et al.: Association between depressive symptoms and serum concentrations of homocysteine in men: a population study. Am. J. Clin. Nutr. 2004; 80: 1574–8.

114   Gilbody, S., et al.: Is low folate a risk factor for depression? A meta analysis and exploration of heterogeneity. J. Epid. Comm. Health.2007; 61: 631–7.

115   Abalan, F., et al.: Frequency of deficiencies of vitamin B_{12} and folic acid in patients admitted to a geriatric psychiatry unit. Encephale 1984; 10: 9–12.

116   Kivela, S., et al.: Depression in the aged: Relation to folate and vitamin C, B6. Biol. Psychiatry 1989; 26: 209–213.

117   Wyatt, K., et al. Efficacy of vitamin B_6 in the treatment of PMS: Systematic review. BMJ 1999; 318: 1375–1381.

118   Pilar, S.: Amelioration of premenstrual depressive symptomatology with L-Tryptophan. J Psychiatry and Neuroscience. 1994; 19: 114–119

119 Krahwinkel, M., et al.: Positionspapier der DGE. Strategien zur Verbesserung der Folatversorgung in Deutschland. DGE. 2006; 12.
120 US Departement of Agriculture. National food consumption survey. 1986.
121 Souccar, T., Curtay, J.P.: Le nouveau -guide des vitamines. Edition Seuil. 1996; 11–12.
122 Dupin, et al.: Apports nutritionels conseillés pour la population française. Paris: Tec & Doc Lavoisier 1992; 2.
123 Guilland: Évaluation de l'apport alimentaire vitaminique en Bourgogne. Ann. -Nutr. Metabol. 1986; 30: 21–46.
124 Hercberg: Consommation alimentaire d'un echantillon représentatif de la popula-tion du Val de Marne. Rev. Epidémiol Santé Publ. 1991; 39: 245–261.
125 Why Top Doctors Take Supplements. Prevention 1994; (2).
126 Kallmann, B.: Micronutrient intakes in laboratory animals and humans. J. Applied Nutr. 1989; 41: 23–25.
127 Dietl, H., Ohlenschläger, G.: Handbuch der Orthomolekularen Medizin. 1994; 26–28.
128 Hu, F., Rimm, E., Stampfer, M., et al.: Frequent nut consumption and the risk of coronary heart disease in women: prospective cohort study. BMJ 1998; 317: 1341–1345.
129 Fraser, G. E., et al.: A possible protective effect of nut consumption on the risk of coronary heart disease. The adventist health study. Arch. Int. Med. 1992; 152: 1416–1424.
130 Prineas, R.J., Kushi, L.H., et al.: Walnuts and serum lipids. N. Engl. J. Med. 1993; 329: 359.
131 Ohlenschläger, G.: Handbuch der Orthomolekularen Medizin. Heidelberg: Haug 1994; 111–112.
132 Kahaly, G., et al.: Cost estimation of thyroid disorders in Germany. Thyroid. 2002; 12: 909–14.
133 Pietrzik, K.: Modern Lifestyle, Lower Energy Intake and Micronutrient Status. Berlin: Springer 1991; 103–114.
134 Brockert, S.: Vital 1985; 3: 63ff.
135 Guilland, J.C., et al.: Influence de modalités de cuisson sur la perte en thiamine, en riboflavine, et en niacine de la viande de boeuf. In: Bernard, A., et al.: Aspects nutritionels des constituant des aliments. ENS.BANA, Dijon/TEC. DOC, Paris 1992; 217–226.
136 Schünke, Kuhlmann, Lau: Orthomolekulare Medizin. Bio Medoc Verlag 1991; 24.
137 Curtay, J.P.: La Nutrithérapie. Bases Scientifique et Pratique Médicale. Paris: Edi-tions Boirons 1995; 54–55.
138 Chemische Qualitätssicherung der Krankenhauskost. Akut Ernähr. Med. 1993; 18: 296–304.
139 Mareschi: Valeur calorique de l'alimentation et couverture des apports nutritionnels conseillés en vitamines de l'homme adulte. Ann. Nutr. Metab. 1984; l 28: 11–23.
140 Hulshof: Is food variety conductive to a more adequate diet? Assessment of variety, dutch clustering and adaquacy of eating patterns. CIP Data Koninklijke Bibliotheek, La Haye 1993.
141 Dietl, H., Gesche, M.: Herzaktive Nährstoffe. Spitta Verlag 1999; 200.
142 GFK-Ernährungsforschung: Nationale Verzehrsstudie 1985–1989.
143 DGE Aktuell vom 23.10.1997.
144 Basu, Schorah: Vitamin C in Health and Diseases. Westport: Avery Publishing 1982; 84–85.
145 Enstrom, Kanim, Klein: Vitamin C in-take and mortality among a sample of the United States population. Epidemi-ology 1992; 3(3): 194–202.
146 Pyor: The Free Radical Chemistry of Cigarette Smoke and the Inactivation of Alpha-1-Proteinase Inhibitor. In: Taylor (ed.): Pulmonary Emphysema and Proteolysis. New York: Academic Press 1986; 369–392.
147 Deutsche Gesellschaft für Ernährung. Ernährungsbericht 2000. S. 316.
148 Giovanucci, E.: Tomatoes, tomato based products, lycopene and cancer: review of epidemiological evidence: J Nat Cancer Inst 1999; 91: 317–331.
149 Yong, L., et al: Intake of vitamin E, C and A and the risk of lung cancer. The NHANES epidemiologic follow up study. Am J Epidemiol 1997; 146: 231–243.
150 Voorrips, L., et al.: A propective cohort study on antioxidants and folate intake and male lung cancer risk. Cancer Epid. Bio. Prev. 2000; 9: 357–65.
151 Hongbing, S., et al.: Dietary folate and Lung cancer risk in former smokers. A case control study. Cancer Epid. Bio. Prev. 2003; 12: 980–986.
152 Hennekens, C., Stampfer J., et al.: Lack of effect of long term supplementation with beta carotin on the incidence of malignant neoplasms and cardiovascular disease. N Engl J Med 1996; 334: 1145–1149.
153 Willett, W., et al.: Plasma folate, vitamin B$_6$, vitamin B$_{12}$, homocysteine, and risk of breast cancer. J. Natl. Cancer Inst. 2003; 95: 373–80.
154 Giovanucci, E., et al.: Vitamin B$_6$ intake, alcohol consumption, and colorectal cancer: a longitudinal

population based cohort of women. Gastroenterology. 2005; 128: 1830–1837.

155   Giovanucci, E., et al.: Alcohol, low methionine-low folate diets, and risk of colon cancer in men. J. Natl. Cancer Inst. 1995; 87: 265–73.

156   Palan, et al.: Effects of Smoking and Oral Contraceptives on Plasma Carotin Levels in Healthy Women. Am. J. Obst. Gynecol. 1989; 161: 881–885.

157   He, J., et al.: Increased consumption of fruit and vegetable is related to a reduced risk of coronary heart disease: meta-analysis of cohort studies. J. Hum. Hypertens. 2007; 21: 717–28.

158   Biesalski, H., et al.: Beta-Carotine supplementation and sun induced biochem-ical alterations of the human skin. International Symposium on Antioxidants and disease prevention. Stockholm: ILSI 1993; 88.

159   Stähelin, H.: Senile dementia in relation to nutritional factors: Bibl. Nutr. et Dieta 1986; 38: 136–144.

160   Yao, Y., et al.: Decline of serum cobalmin levels with increasing age among geriatric patients. Arch. Med.1994; 3:

161   Pennix, B., et al.:Vitamin B_{12} deficiency and depression in physically disabled older women: epidemiologic evidence from the Women's Health and Aging Study. Am. J. Psychiatry. 2000; 157: 715–21.

162   Tiermeier, T., et al.: Vitamin B_{12}, Folate, and Homocysteine and Depression: The Rotterdam Study. Am. J. Psychiatry. 2002; 159: 2099–2101.

163   Pittas, A., et al.: Vitamin D and Kalzium intake in relation to type 2 diabetes in women. Diabetes Care. 2006; 29: 650–6.

164   Colditz, et al.:Diet and risk of clinical diabetes. Am. J. Clin. Nutr. 1992; 55: 14–20.

165   Folsom, A., et al.: Serum and dietary mag-nesium and the risk of type 2 diabetes. Arch. Intern. Med. 1999; 159: 2110–20.

166   Kushi, L., et al.: Carbohydrates, dietary fiber and the incidence of type 2 diabetes in older women. Am. J. Clin. Nutr. 2000: 71: 921–30.

167   Melnick, S., et al.: Association of serum and dietary magnesium with cardiovas-cular disease, hypertension and diabetes. J. Clin. Epid. 1996; 48: 927–40.

168   Davie, Gold, et al.: Effect of Vitamin C on Glycosylation of Proteins. Diabetes 1992; 41: 167–173.

169   Poalisso, et al.: Metabolic benefits de-riving from chronic vitamin C supplementa-tion in aged non-insulin dependent diabetics. J. Am. Coll. Nutr. 1995; 14: 387–392.

170   Barringer, T., et al. Effect of a multivitamin and mineral supplement on infection and quality of life. A randomized, double blind, placebo controlled trial. An. Intern. Med. 2003; 138: 365–371.

171   Döll, M.: Körperliche Belastung und sportliche Aktivität – erhöhter oxidativer Stress durch freie Radikale. Journal für Orthomolekulare Medizin 1996; 4: 316–319.

172   Neue Nachweismethoden für DNA-Schäden – Zellkerndefekte durch Leistungssport. In: Zeitung für Umweltmedizin. 1994; 4: 8–11.

173   Ohlenschläger, G.: Handbuch der Orthomolekularen Medizin. Haug 1994; 42–43.

174   Henrotte, J.: Genetic regulation of blood and tissue magnesium content. Magnesium 1988; 7: 306–314.

175   Grundy, S., et al.: Influence of nicotinic acid on metabolism of cholesterol and triglycerides in man. J. Lipid. Res. 1981; 22: 24–36.

176   Canner, P., et al.: Fifteen year mortality in coronary heart project patients: Long term benefit with niacin. J. Am. Coll. Cardiol. 1986, 8: 1245–1255.

177   Illingworth, et al.: Comparative effects of Lovastatin and Niacin in primary hypercholesterolemia. Arch. Int. Med. 1994; 154: 1586.

178   Ravnskow, U.: Cholesterol lowering trials in coronary heart diseases. Brit. Med. J. 1992; 15: 305.

179   Armstrong, E., et al.: Cost-effectiveness of simavastatin and lovastatin/extended release niacin to achieve LDL and HDL goal using NHANES data. J. Manag. Care Pharm. 2004; 10: 251–70.

180   Bays, H., et al.: Comparison of once daily niacin ET/lovastatin with standard doses of atorvastatin and simavastatin. Am. J. Card. 2003; 15: 667–72.

181   Block, K., et al.: Impact of antioxidant supplementation on chemotherapeutic efficacy: a systematic review of the evidence from randomized controlled trials. Cancer Treat. Rev. 2007; 33: 407–18.

182   Köstler,   W.:   Immunologische   und   spektralanalytische   Veränderungen   durch Quecksilbermobilisierung aus Amalgamfüllungen. Erfahrungsheilkunde 1990; 10: 572–577.

183   Gerhard, I., et al.: Schadstoffe und Fertilitätsstörungen. Schwermetalle und Mineralstoffe. Zentralblatt für Gynäkologie 1992; 114, 593–602.

184   Tikkiwal, M., et al: Effect of zinc administration on seminal zinc and fertility of oligospermic males. Ind. J. Physiol. Pharmacol. 1987; 31, 30–34.

185   Netter, A., et al.: Effects of zinc administration on plasma testosterone and sperm count. Arch. Androl. 1981; 7: 69–73.
186   Daunderer, M.: Handbuch der Amalgamvergiftung. Landsberg: Ecomed, 1992.
187   Wenstrup, D., et al.: Trace element imbalances in isolated subcellular fractions of Alzheimer's disease brains. Brain Research 1990; 533: 125–131.
188   Gebhardt, A., et al.: Bestimmung von Kupfer, Zink, Selen und Quecksilber im Blut von MS Patienten. Laboratoriumsmedizin 1994; 3.
189   Bellinger, D.: Internationaler Kongreß der Umweltmedizin Duisburg. 23.-26. 2.1994.
190   Kuklinsky, B.: Oxidativer Stress in einer Computerzentrale. Zeitung für Umweltmedizin 1997; 1: 42–44.
191   Patel, B., et al.: Dietary antioxidants and asthma in adults. Thorax. 2006; 61: 388–93.
192   Hatch, et al.: Asthma, inhaled antioxidants and dietary antioxidants. Am. J. Clin. Nutr. 1995; 61: 625S-630S.
193   Mineraloscop 1994; 3: 1–2.
194   Andersen, O., et al.: Effects of selenium supplementation on whole body, blood and organ levels of toxic metals in mice. Environ. Health Perspect. 1994; 102 -(suppl. 3): 321–324.
195   Dawson, E., et al.: The effect of ascorbic acid supplementation on the blood lead levels of smokers. J. Am. Col. Nutr. 1999; 18: 166–70.
196   Simon, J.: Relationship of ascorbic acid to blood lead levels. JAMA. 1999; 281: 2340–2.
197   Kuklinsky, B.: Oxidativer Stress in einer Computerzentrale. Zeitung für Umweltmedizin 1997; 1: 42–44.
198   Shrimpton, D.: A scientific evaluation for safe range of intakes. Safety report. EHPM 1997.

Overview of Vitamins

Vitamin	Function	Deficiency symptom**	Therapeutic or preventive use**
Fat soluble vitamins			
Vitamin A (Retinol)	Strong antioxidant; vision; gene transcription; immune function, reproduction; bone metabolism; healthy skin; important for all mucous membranes (eye, mouth, intestines etc.)	Warning: fat soluble vitamins can be overdosed. Watch upper limit. Night blindness (poor vision in dim light); dry eyes; dry hair; dry, rough, scaly, skin; bumpy skin due to buildup of cellular debris in the hair follicles especially on upper arms; brittle nails; growth retardation in children; lowered resistance to infection; low antibody response; low T-cell count; decreased resistance against bacteria of mucosal lining (barrier function) of respiratory tract, gastro-intestinal tract, urinary tract and bladder; rapid weight loss; loss of smell, taste or appetite.	Cataract; dry eyes; infertility; acne
Beta Carotene (Provitamin A)	Is metabolized into vitamin A if needed thus overlapping functions with vitamin A; strong antioxidant; important retina pigment in the eye	Premature cataract formation and macular degeneration; higher oxidative stress	Prevention of free radical diseases (cancer, cardiovascular disease, cataracts, macular degeneration); reduces skin rashes due to sun exposure; skin protection
Vitamin D (Calciferol)	Many hormone - like functions; maintenance of calcium level; bone and teeth formation; brain cell growth; stimulates production of insulin; regulates inflammatory response; immune function, vitamin D receptor is expressed on most immune cells; regulation of blood pressure	Warning: fat soluble vitamins can be overdosed. Watch upper limit. Not really a vitamin but a hormone. Produced by the skin when exposed to sun. Wide spread deficiencies during winter time. Most researched vitamin in the last years. Osteoporosis, osteopenia; immune deficiency; mental decline; rickets; rheumatoid arthritis; low blood calcium level	Prevention of several cancers (colorectal, breast, prostate); osteoporosis, dementia, mental decline; diabetes; asthma; autoimmune diseases; immune deficiency

Vitamin	Function	Deficiency symptom**	Therapeutic or preventive use**
Vitamin E (Tocopherol)	Powerful antioxidant; protects cell membranes and essential fatty acids from free radicals; immune function; red blood cell formation; fertility	High oxidative stress; muscular wasting; anemia, infertility; heart disease; weak immune system	Prevention of cardiovascular disease; prevention of vascular dementia and Alzheimer's

Water soluble vitamins

Vitamin	Function	Deficiency symptom**	Therapeutic or preventive use**
Vitamin C (Ascorbic Acid)	Involved in over 15,000 different metabolic reactions! Strong antioxidant; regenerates other antioxidants like vitamin E; essential for immune function; production of connective tissue and collagen (tendons, blood vessels); production of hormones; wound healing; synthesis of neurotransmitters; synthesis of carnitin for optimal fat burning; etc. etc. etc.	Deferred wound healing; gingivitis, bleeding gums; easy bruising; dry, brittle hair; immune deficiency; dry, rough scaly skin; anemia; fatigue, lethargy, muscle weakness; atherosclerosis	Protection of free radical diseases (cataracts, macular degeneration, cancer, cardiovascular disease); Preventive against atherosclerosis and stroke; hypertension; improves immune function; allergies and asthma due to vitamin C's antihistaminic properties; diabetes; wound healing; chronic fatigue symptom
Vitamin B₁ (Thiamine)	Nerve- and muscle metabolism; carbohydrate metabolism; production of neurotransmitters	Forgetfulness, confusion, irritability, depression, memory problems, disturbed sleep – due to disturbed neurotransmitter production; fatigue, loss of sensation (numbness) in hands and legs; pin-and-needle sensation; heart abnormalities (palpitations); gastrointestinal disorders; constipation; Crohn's disease; recurrent sores (aphthous or oral ulcers); stunted growth; Beriberi (excessive fatigue or muscular weakness. This severe deficiency is uncommon today except in severe alcoholics)	Diabetes; neurological diseases, Alzheimer's, dementia; if deficient vitamin B₁ can optimize brain function, learning capacity, mental alertness, memory and fight depression
Vitamin B₂ (Riboflavin)t	Part of over 60 enzymes of the fat-, carbohydrate- and protein metabolism; energy production; transmission of light signals to the eye; regenerates the important antioxidant glutathione	Fatigue, visual disturbances (light sensitivity, loss of acuity); burning and itching eyes, lips mouth; cracking lips and corners of the mouth; seborrheic dermatitis; brittle hair and fingernails	Migraine; prevention of cataracts; skin disorders

Vitamin	Function	Deficiency symptom**	Therapeutic or preventive use**
Vitamin B$_3$ (Niacin)	Energy metabolism; regulation of blood sugar; cholesterol- and carbohydrate metabolism; functioning of nervous system	The amino acid tryptophan can be metabolized into Vitamin B$_3$. Thus you rarely measure B$_3$ deficiency. However, B$_3$ deficiency can create a shortage of tryptophan which is the building block and limiting factor for the mood enhancing neurotransmitter serotonin. The consequences: depression, sleep disturbances, irritability, anxiety, forgetfulness, memory problems; dry, cracked, scaly skin; dermatitis; muscular weakness; fatigue; loss of appetite	Blood lipid reduction (LDL, triglycerides and increase of HDL); diabetes
Vitamin B$_5$ (Pantothenic Acid)	Utilization of fats, carbohydrates, protein; energy production; production of adrenal- and steroid hormones; production of red blood cells; wound healing; neurotransmitter production; transmission of nerve impulses; production of skin and hair pigments	Chronic fatigue; depression, irritability, insomnia; migraine; lackluster and premature grey hair; impaired wound healing; impaired immunity; burning pain in feet due to problems of nerve conduction	-
Vitamin B$_6$ (Pyridoxine)	Needed to synthesize all protein structures: cellular multiplication and cell repair, proliferation of immune cells, synthesis of hormones and neurotransmitters	Depression, irritability, memory problems, lowered concentration, disturbed sleep, mood swings, mood abnormalities, PMS (premenstrual symptoms) – all of which relate to impaired neurotransmitter production (serotonin, dopamine, melatonin, norepinephrine etc.); neurologic symptoms; migraine; nausea and morning sickness during pregnancy; immune deficiency, susceptibility to infection due to impaired production of immune cells during infection; glucose intolerance; eczema, dermatitis, seborrhea, cracking or sores on lips because skin cells replicate quickly and thus are affected first even by minor vitamin-B$_6$ deficiency; inflammation of mucous membranes of the mouth or tongue; chronic fatigue; muscle weakness	Depression, mood disorders, neurological symptoms; immune deficiency; diabetes; PMS; osteoporosis; nausea during pregnancy; lowers homocysteine and thereby reduces cardiovascular disease, heart attack, strokes and dementia; prevention of several types of cancer; immune deficiency

Vitamin	Function	Deficiency symptom**	Therapeutic or preventive use**
Biotin	Utilization of fats, carbohydrates and amino acids; cellular multiplication	Manufactured by the gut bacteria. Deficiencies are rare. Dry, scaly skin around the eye, nose, mouth; seborrheic dermatitis, brittle nails and dry hair, hair loss	-
Folate / Folic Acid	Cellular division and cell repair; DNA synthesis and repair; development of nervous system of the fetus; lowers homocysteine in the blood; production of neurotransmitters; red blood cell formation; functioning of the brain	Most common vitamin deficiency. Folate is extremely sensitive to destruction by light, oxygen and heat. Alcohol, many prescription drugs and estrogen impair folate-metabolism. Birth defects, low birth weight, premature infants; arteriosclerosis, heart attacks, strokes, dementia due to high homocysteine levels; depression, irritability, mood abnormalities, concentration problems, insomnia due to impaired neurotransmitter production; anemia	All women before menopause to lower the risk of birth defects (neural tube defects); lowers homocysteine reducing cardiovascular disease, heart attacks, strokes, dementia and osteoporosis; prevention of several types of cancer (breast-, ovarian-, prostate-, lung-, colorectal cancer); depression, mood disorders, neurological symptoms; Alzheimer's; immune deficiency
Vitamin B_{12} (Cobalmin)	Synthesis of DNA; production of neurotransmitters; red blood cells, insulation of nerve cells; signal conduction of nerve cells	Deficient most often in elderly as vitamin B_{12} is less absorbed from food. Mainly in the elderly: depression, irritability, memory problems, lowered concentration, disturbed sleep, mood abnormalities, neurologic symptoms, confusion, disorientation, impaired cognitive function, dementia; associated with Alzheimer's; anemia, pale skin, fatigue, weakness; red tongue or mouth; high blood levels of homocysteine; retarded growth	Senile depression, dementia mood disorders, neurologic symptoms; diabetic neuropathy; anemia; AIDS; lowers homocysteine reducing cardiovascular disease, heart attacks, strokes and dementia

** For Disclaimer and Warning see p. 2

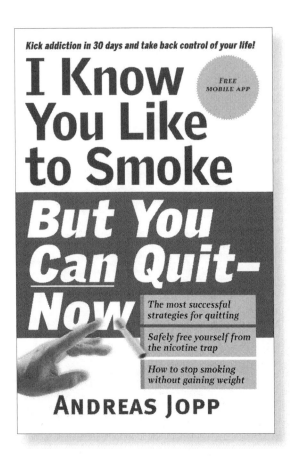

Kick addiction in 30 days and take back control of your life!

I Know You Like to Smoke

FREE MOBILE APP

But You Can Quit—Now

The most successful strategies for quitting

Safely free yourself from the nicotine trap

How to stop smoking without gaining weight

ANDREAS JOPP

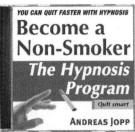

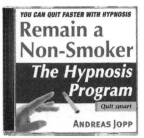

The first CD of the hypnosis program will help you before you quit smoking and on the day you quit. Before quitting, smokers are torn as to whether they will succeed this time or whether they will „miss" something. The hypnosis will give you the deep sense of really doing the right thing.

The second CD of the hypnosis program will help you after you quit smoking. In the first few weeks the addicted brain will always try tointerfere. Here, it is important to continue to keep the access to the subconscious desires open, in order to remain a non-smoker.

37956761R00084

Made in the USA
Middletown, DE
04 March 2019